**Drop All the Pounds You Want
without Giving Up the Foods You Love**

DENISE AUSTIN

WITH AMY CAMPBELL, M.S., R.D., C.D.E.

EAT CARBS, LOSE WEIGHT

RODALE

© 2005 by Denise Austin

Printed in the United States of America
Rodale Inc. makes every effort to use acid-free ♾, recycled paper ♲.

Exercise photographs on pages 86 to 98 by Mary Noble Ours. Photograph on page iii courtesy of the author.
All other photographs by Michael O'Neill.

Book design by Tara Long

Library of Congress Cataloging-in-Publication Data

Austin, Denise.
    Eat carbs, lose weight : drop all the pounds you want without giving up the foods you love /
Denise Austin, with Amy Campbell.
        p.   cm.
    Includes index.
    ISBN-13 978–1–59486–233–5 trade hardcover
    ISBN-10 1–59486–233–8 trade hardcover
    1. Reducing diets.   2. Carbohydrates in human nutrition.   I. Campbell, Amy, M.S., R.D., C.D.E.
II. Title.
    RM222.2.A88   2005
    613.2'5—dc22   2005013080

Distributed to the trade by Holtzbrinck Publishers

2 4 6 8 10 9 7 5 3 1 hardcover

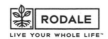

We inspire and enable people to improve their lives and the world around them

For more of our products visit **rodalestore.com** or call 800-848-4735

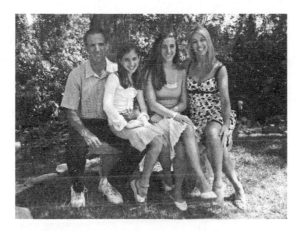

To Jeff, Kelly, and Katie, my true joys in life.

CONTENTS

ACKNOWLEDGMENTS

I'm truly grateful to God for my wonderful family. There's nothing more important to me than their health and happiness. Thanks to my husband, Jeff, who always puts us "girls" first; and to my precious daughters, Kelly and Katie, who are growing up way too fast. I cherish every moment.

To my sweet Mom in heaven, who was my true role model—so incredibly dedicated to all five of us kids. And to my Dad, who taught us perseverance and determination. I've been blessed with three awesome sisters and a great brother. We have so much fun together!

A big thanks to Amy Campbell for her fantastic nutritional expertise, and to Alisa Bauman, who helped "put it all together." Thanks also to my friends at *Prevention* magazine for their support of my monthly fitness column, and to all at Rodale Books, especially Tami Booth Corwin and Mariska Van Aalst. To my agents, Jan Miller and Michael Broussard—I love you guys!

Also, I really want to thank all of my friends at Waterfront Media for making my DeniseAustin.com Web site such a valuable tool for so many women who want to lose weight and feel good about themselves. I love it, and I love what I do—knowing I'm out there helping people.

INTRODUCTION

Finally, an eating plan that allows you to stay fit and healthy forever

If, like me, you love bread, potatoes, and other carbs, the low-carbohydrate dieting craze that has swept the country (and even much of the world) probably has you feeling downright disheartened. That's certainly how I felt after I kept hearing about the wonders of low-carb diets from my girlfriends, news reports, advertisements, and even some of my fans.

I have always believed in the goodness of carbohydrates, but after hearing so much about low-carb diets, I began to investigate it myself. Like you, I want to feel and look my best. I need to. It's part of my job. I'm in front of millions of fans every day for my television show. I *have* to look and feel my best. So, not long ago, I decided to give a low-carb diet a try.

I lasted one day. Almost as soon as I stopped eating carbs, I found I wanted them even more. I daydreamed about biting into a chunk of whole-grain bread with butter and about popping a potato into the microwave. Worse, I felt tired. I didn't have the get-up-and-go that I was used to. My energy is important to me. I exercise most mornings and try to get a lot done during the day. When I pick my daughters up from school, I like to greet them with a happy and hearty hello and feel up to whatever activity they suggest we do for the rest of the day with zest. On my one-day-long low-carb diet, however, I just didn't feel like myself. Rather than exercise, I wanted to take a nap. Instead of work,

I wanted to watch television. It wasn't the me I was used to. It wasn't the me I wanted to be.

I wasn't willing to sacrifice that much just to look great. I knew there had to be a better way. I've always felt that *feeling* good goes hand in hand with *looking* good. I decided right then and there that I would search for an eating plan that allowed me—and my friends and fans—to eat carbs and not gain weight.

I went straight to the top, to the most well-respected health center in the country—Harvard! My search took me to Amy Campbell, M.S., R.D., C.D.E., one of the leading nutritionists in the country. During her 16 years as a registered dietitian and nutrition educator at Harvard-affiliated Joslin Diabetes Center in Boston, Amy has helped thousands of people with diabetes lose weight and keep it off—without giving up carbs!

I sought out Amy's advice. I told her that I needed carbs in my diet. Carbs gave me the energy to be me. Plus, I loved them. I told her, "I want to eat my carbs and look great, too." Amy helped me to develop the revolutionary eating plan that you will find in this book. Not only does it include carbs, it includes all of my favorite carbs: pudding, bread, potatoes, even cheesecake. Not only did I not *gain* weight on this plan, I *lost* weight! I also felt more energetic and definitely more satisfied. I enjoyed every delicious meal I ate without guilt. I noticed no cravings or between-meal hunger pains. It was truly amazing, and I couldn't wait to share the news with my sisters, girlfriends, and fans.

DELICIOUS, SATISFYING, AND HEALTHY

I love whole-grain bread, the kind made with molasses and smeared with a touch of butter. Low-carb diets tell you to stay away from pineapple, bananas, oranges, and cherries. Not me. I love these foods. These foods are so good for you. I'm not about to give them up.

You shouldn't either. I'm excited to tell you that you *can* have your carbs and lose weight, too. I've always believed that healthy carbs are an important part of every healthy eating plan. Not only are they a vital source of energy and stamina, they also help fight cancer, heart disease, and, yes, even diabetes!

Ever since I began my health and fitness career more than 25 years ago, I've been preaching the benefits of eating balanced portions of carbohydrates, proteins, and fats. I've said that *all* of those nutrients should be included in a healthy diet. I've *always* believed in balance—and so do the doctors, nutritionists, and scientists that I talk to on a regular basis.

That said, the eating plan you will find in this book is *not* the same low-fat, high-carbohydrate eating plan that I—and many others—followed during the 1980s and 1990s. It's quite revolutionary, as you will soon see. On this plan, you will eat the *right* carbs in the *right* amounts for optimum health, energy, and weight loss. Those low-fat, high-carbohydrate diets that were popular during the 1980s and 1990s included too much of the wrong types of carbs. On the *Eat Carbs, Lose Weight* plan, you will eat carbs in balance with proteins and fats. This will lessen your appetite and rev up your fat-burning furnace.

In addition to the *right* carbs, the *Eat Carbs, Lose Weight* plan includes small portions of some other seemingly decadent foods, such as lean meat and even butter. As with carbs, those foods have been vilified at one time or another by various diets du jour, but neither is bad for you when eaten in moderation. That's the secret to losing weight and loving every taste of it: moderation. If you eat reasonable portions of the foods you love, there's no reason to omit any food—no matter how seemingly decadent—from your diet. I'm living proof!

I enjoy the way I eat. I feel satisfied after every meal and have more energy today than I did at age 20. I believe that life is too short to deprive yourself of your favorite foods. In my mind, there's no greater torture than to see, smell, and even dream about certain foods but never actually allow yourself to taste them. Considering that carbohydrates are a key nutrient that our bodies need, we should listen to our taste buds! Food is fabulous, and you should enjoy it.

MOVE OVER, BACON

If you, too, have tried one low-carb diet—or several—without success, you may wonder if there's something wrong with you. After all, how hard can it be to stick to a diet that includes bacon and burgers?

I can tell you that there is absolutely *nothing* wrong with you. For the past 3 years, I've received tons of mail from fans who tell me they miss their carbs. They desperately want to lose weight, but each time they try to cut out the carbs, they end up craving carbs even more. They yearn to savor the aroma of fresh-baked bread, the crunch of breakfast cereal, and the comfort of a baked potato right out of the oven. They tell me they are sick and tired—literally—from being on low-carb diet plans. They have no energy, they can't concentrate, and they feel irritable. They write things like, "If this is what it takes to lose weight, maybe I'll just stay fat!"

Indeed, as Kristi Toms told me, "I crave my noodles, bread, and rice dishes. I enjoy all veggies and meats, but if I try to cut out the carbs, I tend to crave them and eat more of them than I would if I had just left well enough alone."

Another fan, Ashley Reid, wrote, "The low-carb diet made me feel very tired and very greasy. I felt like I was just putting on the pounds and not attempting to lose them. Plus, I was *always* hungry."

I want you to feel as happy about your food choices as I feel about mine. I want you to be able to savor the taste of bread—or even a cookie—without feeling a smidgen of guilt. I want you to be able to nibble on a bite of any food—really, *any* food—without feeling as if you are going to lose control. I want you to be able to eat in a way—as I do—that not only helps you control your weight but also improves your health, mood, and energy. Finally, I want you to be able to try this way of eating and love it so much that you'll want to stick with it for life—because that's the only way to keep off the weight.

That's right—for life. Unlike with many diets that last 2 weeks, you're about to embark on a lifelong eating plan, one that's good for your health, realistic, simple, and delicious. Call it a diet if you must, but know that once you go on this diet, and see the results, you will want to stay on it for life.

In *Eat Carbs, Lose Weight,* you will also discover a nourishing, delicious, and sound way of eating—one that is healthy for the entire family. That's important, too. Who has time to cook two meals every night: one for you and one for everyone else? I know I don't. That's why my meal choices include wholesome foods that my daughters and husband love as much as I do.

The meal plan in *Eat Carbs, Lose Weight* reflects the food choices I now make every day. It includes all of my favorite foods and none of the foods that I consider unhealthy. For example, I try not to eat any foods with hydrogenated fat. Created during food processing, these fats have been linked to an increased risk of heart disease and cancer. Plus, your body can't burn off these fats like it can other fats. The *Eat Carbs, Lose Weight* meal plan includes very little of this fat. It's as low in hydrogenated fat as a meal plan can possibly get!

The meal plan is also good for you. By that, I mean it's healthy. That's really important when it comes to eating to lose weight. When you are carrying around a lot of extra pounds—or even just a few—in your abdomen, your metabolism doesn't work as efficiently as it would if you were at your healthiest weight. Your blood sugar levels may remain chronically high, for example. Insulin levels may be high as well. You may not technically have diabetes, but you could have something almost as deadly: metabolic syndrome. This cluster of adverse health problems includes low levels of the good HDL cholesterol, high blood pressure, and elevated levels of certain proteins in your blood that raise your risk for heart attack.

Metabolic syndrome and its close relative diabetes have become epidemics in this country and are growing at an alarming rate. Diabetes now affects more than 18 million people. More than a million people are diagnosed with diabetes *every year.* Another 16 million have prediabetes, which means their blood sugar levels are inching upward but are not high enough to be considered full-blown diabetes. Another 47 million people have recognized metabolic syndrome, and many more probably have it but don't even know it

"I Ate Carbs and Lost Weight!"

Name: Karla J. Reynolds

Age: 39

Town: Bloomington, Indiana

Weight Lost: 10 pounds in 4 weeks

Other Accomplishments: Lost 13 inches and looks and feels healthier

"My battle with weight began in college and escalated from there. When I was growing up, my mother always served healthful, well-balanced meals, so my weight stayed steady. But as soon as I moved out, I found it was easier to eat whatever and whenever I wanted, which usually included fast food.

"When I became pregnant with my son, I ballooned to 204 pounds. I took it off a few years later, but only because I was going through a stressful time and wasn't really eating anything at all. Not the best solution.

"When I started eating again, the weight came back on with a vengeance and refused to leave—probably because my metabolism had slowed down from the lack of eating. Then a couple of years ago, I had a hysterectomy, which caused me to gain even more weight.

"To lose the weight, I've tried everything—diet pills, cutting out fats, cutting out break-fast, skipping meals, and fad diets. None of these tactics worked. I would find myself bingeing in the evening because I was so hungry—or at least I thought I was.

"Just as I was beginning to feel as though I'd never take the weight off, I heard about *Eat Carbs, Lose Weight.* Her diet seemed to be the most sensible I've heard of yet, and one that I could get my whole family to participate in as well. Aside from the 10 pounds and 13 inches I lost, what I liked the most about the program was the way it affected my energy level and the way I feel about myself. I now have energy to spare, and I don't get that incredibly tired feeling after lunch. I look and feel healthier, and my cravings have become almost nonexistent. My clothes fit more loosely now, and I'm more motivated to exercise than ever.

"I knew the diet was paying off when one of my coworkers said, 'You're looking svelte these days,' and my husband commented that I looked healthier and thinner.

"This eating plan has been one of the best things to happen to me and my family. It is easy to follow, and the recipes are easy to prepare and taste fantastic. Thanks, Denise!"

Karla's advice: "Get the temptation foods out of the house and follow the meal plans. Food becomes less of an issue if you know you can snack during the day."

because their blood sugar levels remain just below their doctors' radar. (All together, that's 81 million people—over 27 percent of the total population, or one in four people!)

Sadly, diabetes is also becoming more common in children. About 210,000 children now have diabetes. Children as young as age 4 are now being diagnosed with type 2 diabetes, once considered "adult-onset diabetes" because it rarely developed before adulthood.

Blood sugar problems raise your risk for just about every disease and health problem imaginable, from eye disease to heart disease to cancer. So, you can see why I think losing weight in a healthful way is so important. Even if you have not been diagnosed with metabolic syndrome, prediabetes, or diabetes itself, your metabolism may not be working as efficiently as it should. Weight loss will help, but to increase your chances of living a long, happy, and healthy life, you should lose weight in the healthiest way possible.

Many people erroneously believe that diabetes is caused by eating too much sugar. This is a myth, says nutritionist Amy Campbell. Type 2 diabetes may be caused by many factors, but the two most common are too little exercise and too many calories. Amy's nutrition suggestions not only have helped thousands of people with prediabetes and diabetes get in control of their blood sugar but also have allowed them to lose weight, increase their energy, and boost their mood—all while eating the foods they love. That's why her insights into the meal plans for this book were so critical. With Amy's help, I've made sure that the *Eat Carbs, Lose Weight* meal plan is healthy for everyone—even people with diabetes.

A DIET THAT YOU'LL LOVE FOR A LIFETIME

Amy and I both agree that no diet is worth the effort if it forces you to eat foods you don't like and omit foods that you love. That's why we made sure the *Eat Carbs, Lose Weight* meal plan includes a variety of delicious foods. I'm confident you will love every bite of every day of the plan.

With *Eat Carbs, Lose Weight*, you will welcome your favorite foods—real bread, hearty pasta dishes, and even potatoes—back to the dinner table and still lose all the pounds you want—for good. Each day, you will be eating healthful meals that include plenty of vegetables, whole grains, and lean protein foods such as pork tenderloin and chicken breast. You'll also be able to savor plenty of sweet tastes from fruit, pudding, cookies, and more. How can you eat so many seemingly decadent foods and still lose weight? The secret lies in the following guiding principles.

✧ Three meals and two snacks—every day. As you will soon learn, eating every 3 to 4 hours is critical to your weight-loss success. It will help stabilize blood sugar levels, which, in turn, will elevate your mood and energy levels and drive down cravings and appetite.

✧ A 50–25–25 mix of carbohydrates to protein and fat. Amy and I believe that this is the ideal formula for weight loss and good health. This allows you to eat the carbs you love without overeating. You'll lose weight, reduce your cravings, and boost your energy levels.

✧ A focus on quality, wholesome foods. Too often in our harried and hurried world, many of us rely on processed foods for most of our nutrition. Although not all processed foods are bad for you, some of them are packed with disease-promoting hydrogenated fats and hunger-producing refined sugars. The meal plan in this book focuses on the best of what Mother Nature has to offer: fruits, vegetables, whole grains, and lean protein sources such as chicken breast. These foods provide the fiber and wholesome nutrition you need to turn down hunger, stabilize blood sugar, and stay satisfied.

✧ A daily dose of decadence. If you've been on many diets, then you know that deprivation doesn't work. When you feel guilty and try not to eat your favorite foods, you will want them even more. That's why the meal plan in this book includes sweet tastes from desserts like Apple Crumble with Oat Crust and Peach Melba, among many other sweet foods. You'll also find out how to substitute your favorite, most decadent food for these suggested desserts.

In addition to the meal plan, *Eat Carbs, Lose Weight* includes some exercise. I wouldn't be Denise Austin if I didn't suggest at least *some* exercise, right? Although some popular diets out there suggest that you can lose weight through dietary changes alone—and not by adding any exercise—I just don't buy it. When you lose weight by cutting calories and not taking part in any exercise, you tend to lose it from both your fat and your muscle stores. This only sets you up for failure later on. Your muscles help to power your metabolism. Each pound of muscle burns 35 to 50 calories a day just to maintain itself. Plus, muscles throughout your body burn many, many more calories every time they move. Dieting without exercise slows your metabolism. It's that simple.

Dieting *with* exercise does the reverse. As you build and sculpt lean muscle tissue, you'll increase your metabolism. New research has found that after an exercise session, your metabolism stays elevated for up to 13 hours!

Daily doses of exercise also help to control appetite. They also boost your mood, making you less likely to binge when under stress. And exercise burns off excess calories and helps control insulin levels. If you want to live a long and healthy life, you *must* exercise.

The exercise plan in this book is quick and simple. My Daily Dozen routine includes just 12 moves a day for a total of 12 minutes. That's it! This fit-forever routine includes a blend of my favorite yoga, Pilates, and strength moves. You'll work every muscle in your body as you jump-start your metabolism. It's a very efficient 12 minutes of toning. Do you have 12 minutes for slimmer thighs? A slimmer waistline? Firmer arms? Do you have 12 minutes for better health and a faster metabolism? Yes, you do. You can do it!

A SNEAK PREVIEW

I'm so excited to share with you this revolutionary way of eating. I can't wait until you embark on the *Eat Carbs, Lose Weight* journey and begin to eat delicious and fabulous foods *every day*. I'm willing to bet that you are just as excited. You're going to shed up to 8 pounds this month (maybe even more!), and you'll lose a dress size in just 4 weeks. Stick with it and you'll lose all the weight you want, you'll keep it off, and you won't have to give up any of your favorite foods to make it happen.

I love food, and I love eating. Throughout the pages of *Eat Carbs, Lose Weight,* I'm going to teach you my secrets to losing weight, keeping it off, and loving every taste of it. You will make smarter food choices—more delicious food choices. In *Eat Carbs, Lose Weight,* you will embark on a 4-week eating plan that will guide you in a healthful way of enjoying savory, crunchy, energy-boosting carbs. Through *Eat Carbs, Lose Weight,* you will . . .

Reduce your cravings.

Boost your metabolism.

Lessen your appetite.

Rev up your energy.

And, most important of all, lose the weight for life.

You'll stay fit and healthy forever!

In part 1, you'll explore your relationship with carbohydrates. This is the meat and potatoes behind the meal plan, if you will. It's important that you read these chapters. They will help you to understand how the meal plan works and why various foods are included. They will arm you with the knowledge you need for optimum success. Here you'll learn how to eat the right carbs in the right amounts. You'll find out what really causes carbohydrate addiction and how to avoid it without cutting carbs. You'll also discover what foods set off cravings and how to satisfy your cravings without bingeing. Finally, I'll let you in on which carbs help you look and feel your best.

In part 2, you'll find the *Eat Carbs, Lose Weight* meal plan. It's delicious, it's simple, and it's healthy. You will love it.

In part 3, you'll find the *Eat Carbs, Lose Weight* recipe collection. Here you'll find more than 90 all-new recipes. These meals really hit the spot!

Once you've read and understood all of part 1, you're ready to start your *Eat Carbs, Lose Weight* lifestyle. I hope your taste buds are ready, because you will be eating so many delicious meals. In addition to some of the healthiest foods on the planet, you'll also be savoring some Coffee-Chocolate Waffles, Fruity Ginger Smoothies, and a trail mix with chocolate chips, among many other wonderful foods.

My mouth is watering. How about yours? This truly simple, easy, and healthy way of eating will help you to shed pounds quickly while you reduce cravings, boost energy, and feel more satisfied after every meal. Turn to chapter 1 and start your delicious weight-loss journey today!

The Method behind the Meal Plan

Part 1 of the book is so important that I'd like to explore this section in more detail.

In chapter 1, you'll learn why low-fat diets *and* low-carb diets have only made Americans fatter. Here, you'll discover why a balanced eating plan that includes a 50-25-25 breakdown of carbohydrates to protein and fat is so critical to your weight-loss success.

In chapter 2, you'll find out why eating carbohydrates is essential for weight loss and optimum health. From lowering your appetite to boosting your mood and energy, there are many compelling reasons to put carbs back on your plate.

In chapter 3, you'll read all about carbohydrate addiction. If you have ever felt out of control when you've seen or smelled a certain carbohydrate food—whether it was a piece of cake or a warm dinner roll—you are not alone. You'll learn why you find carbs so tempting, as well as effective ways to regain control of your eating. Once you've put the advice in this chapter to work for you, you'll be able to nibble on a bite or two of a chocolate chip cookie without going overboard.

In chapter 4, you'll find four smart-carb strategies that will help reduce your cravings, improve your energy, lower your appetite, and much more. Once you understand these smart-carb strategies, I can help you design your own smart-carb meals.

Chapter 5 will introduce you to the *Eat Carbs, Lose Weight* fitness plan. These 12 moves will sculpt sexy muscles and boost your metabolism long term.

In chapter 6, you'll learn how the *Eat Carbs, Lose Weight* diet works. You'll find out how we chose certain foods for the meal plan—and how you can make smart substitutes when needed.

Finally, in chapter 7, you'll discover everything you need to know to stick with the *Eat Carbs, Lose Weight* plan long term. From eating out at restaurants to surviving the holidays with your family, you'll learn effective tips for staying in control and reducing cravings and diet sabotage.

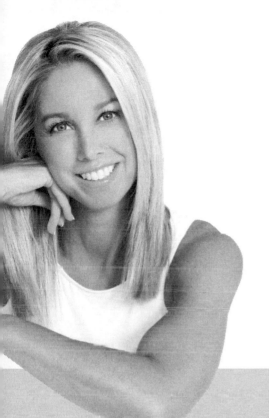

PART 1

Your Relationship with Carbs

TIME FOR A NEW APPROACH

Low-fat diets and low-carb diets have only made Americans fatter—there's a better way

Today you need not travel far to see and hear about the so-called evils of carbohydrates, better known as "carbs." In the grocery store, you encounter food product after food product that claims to be "low in carbs" or "carb smart." On television, you see commercials that depict good-intentioned dieters who are counting their carbs and—in the name of good health and weight loss—switching from a diet rich in bread, pasta, and rice to one that includes fried chicken, steak, and other protein foods. At work, restaurants, and social settings, you probably overhear conversations about how people are cutting their carbs in order to lose weight. For example, someone might say, "Oh no, waiter, no bread for me. I'm trying to be good today."

Are carbs really the cause of all of our dieting problems? Does a diet rich in carbs promote weight gain, heart disease, and diabetes, as many low-carb dieters believe?

I have never believed it, and my coauthor, Amy Campbell, M.S., R.D., C.D.E., of the Harvard-affiliated Joslin Diabetes Center, has always answered those questions with a definitive "no." I've always had faith in the importance of carbs. For many years, I've looked to carbs to keep my energy levels up and my weight down. When I was a young athlete who competed in gymnastics, my coaches often preached the benefits of carbs. Carbs equaled energy, they told us. Later, when I became a television and video fitness host, carbs helped me to find the energy to film multiple programs in a single day.

But in the last couple of years, when I turned 45, it was becoming more difficult to control my weight. So I started eating all the right carbs, and it made a difference.

So that led to the creation of the revolutionary *Eat Carbs, Lose Weight* eating plan. I met with Amy and asked her to help me design an eating plan that included carbs but allowed me and my friends and fans to maintain weight. Instead, she developed a revolutionary eating plan that included the best of both the high-carbohydrate, low-fat diets of the 1980s and 1990s and the low-carbohydrate diets of the new millennium but removed the unhealthy fats, deprivation, between-meal hunger, and cravings. And to our delight, the diet helped us lose all the weight we wanted and keep it off—for good!

Almost everyone Amy counsels with type 2 diabetes needs to lose weight. Indeed, as Amy says, weight loss is the most important change someone with diabetes can make to normalize blood sugar levels. Does she suggest a low-carb diet full of meat, eggs, and butter? No, she doesn't. Does she suggest a high-carbohydrate, low-fat diet? No, she doesn't do that either.

Rather, Amy suggests a balanced approach that includes moderate amounts of carbohydrates (50 percent of your daily calories), protein, and fat (each 25 percent of your daily calories). Not only do her patients lose weight, they are able to keep it off long term. Their blood sugar stays in check, they feel more energetic, and, most important, they report that they enjoy the food they eat—and their lives.

Amy used that 50–25–25 carbohydrate, protein, and fat formula when she designed the meal plans used in this book. We knew, based on Amy's nearly 20 years of experience in the field of weight loss and diabetes, that the meal plan would work. To ensure that the plan was not only *effective* but also *realistic,* Amy and I tested it on a group of volunteers who visited my Web site seeking answers to their weight-loss problems.

After 4 weeks on the diet, the participants not only lost an average of 8 pounds but also looked better and felt better. They lost inches around their waist and hips, and they enjoyed many flattering compliments from family and friends. They reported feeling more energetic, happier, calmer, sexier, and healthier. That's right, as you will learn in chapter 2, the right carbs in the right amounts do more than help you lose weight. They can help boost your mood as well.

And that's what's really important, isn't it? If you lose weight by cutting carbs, only to feel deprived and cranky, is it worth it? I know it wouldn't be worth it to me. I love nibbling on whole-grain bread. I love rice and muffins and crackers. I love fruit. I'm not willing to give those foods up.

And I don't have to. Neither do you. There is a better way.

HOW CARBS EARNED A BAD REPUTATION

So if a diet that includes your favorite carbohydrate foods can actually promote weight loss and good health, how did carbs earn such a bad reputation? To answer that question, we must take a trip back to the 1980s and 1990s, when carbs were in their heyday.

During these decades, many people were counting and cutting their fat grams in order to lose weight and improve their heart health. Studies had recently shown that a diet high in fat led to heart disease and excess weight. Dieters also knew that fat contained more calories per gram than carbohydrate or protein: 9 calories per gram of fat compared with just 4 for the others. Biochemists were also telling us that the body more efficiently shuttled excess calories from fat into fat cells than it did excess calories from carbs. The body actually had to *burn* calories in order to convert carbohydrates into fat.

With that news, many dieters switched from foods high in fat to foods high in carbs. At breakfast, they traded in their doughnuts for plain bagels. For lunch, they ordered a salad with fat-free dressing rather than burgers and fries. At dinner, they replaced those fatty steaks with pasta and red sauce. Many people did indeed lose weight, but many more gained it back. Some gained back more weight than they lost. During these decades, the average amount of fat that Americans consumed dropped as the numbers of overweight and obese Americans climbed.

The promoters of low-carb diets have blamed this weight gain on the carbs. They say a diet rich in carbs spikes blood sugar levels, causing a sharp rise in the hormone insulin, which is responsible for shuttling sugar into hungry cells, including your fat cells. When insulin rises too quickly, blood sugar drops too quickly, making you hungry and tired. You respond by eating more carbs.

To some extent the logic is true, but it doesn't tell the whole story.

Let's take a look at why people *really* gained weight during the 1980s and 1990s. First, and possibly most important, food manufacturers responded to the low-fat craze by removing the fat from many of their products and, quite often, replacing it with sugar, a type of carbohydrate. Because of the addition of sugar, many low-fat products, including cookies and cakes, were just as high in calories as their full-fat cousins.

Indeed, when researchers at Deakin University in Melbourne, Australia, examined the calorie content of low- and reduced-fat products, they discovered that foods with a "low-fat" or "reduced-fat" claim on the label generally contained more calories per serving than higher-fat vegetable-based dishes such as vegetarian lasagna. The researchers concluded that consuming high-fat vegetarian foods would be better for weight loss than switching to a diet based on low-fat and fat-free products.*

Not only were low-fat foods just as caloric as their higher-fat cousins, many people ate more of these foods because they thought they were "healthy." Think back to those years. Did you dish up two scoops of low-fat ice cream instead of your usual one scoop of the premium variety? Did you not think twice about eating an entire bag of baked potato chips or pretzels—because they were low in fat? How about those fat-free cookies? Did you stick to just one, or did you more likely eat four or five of them at a time?

---

*Although our meal plan in Eat Carbs, Lose Weight *includes meat, it follows some of this logic because it excludes processed low-fat food products. Also, cutting fat in other ways—using less butter when frying foods or trimming fat off your cuts of meat, for instance—will reduce your caloric intake and result in weight loss. It's the commercially prepared processed foods high in sugar that tend to pack on the pounds.*

"I Ate Carbs and Lost Weight!"

Name: Devan Brittain

Age: 35

Town: Mooresville, North Carolina

Weight Lost: 12 pounds in 4 weeks

Other Accomplishments: Lost 15½ inches and improved her mood

"Like many women, I made the mistake of viewing pregnancy as an open invitation to eat whatever I wanted. I also became ill and was on bed rest during my pregnancy, so exercise was out. The result? I gained 80 pounds.

"Every attempt I made at losing the postbaby weight failed. I even joined Weight Watchers and didn't lose any weight. I decided to try *Eat Carbs, Lose Weight* because Denise Austin is such a tried-and-true exercise legend. I remember getting up and working out to Denise on TV when I was in high school. I knew that if she was involved in the program, it had to be great.

"And great it's been. What I love the most is that this diet helped me conquer my sugar habit. I had tried everything to stop eating sugar, but nothing worked. With this diet, however, I didn't even crave it anymore. I've never felt deprived, and I've always felt satisfied. The recipes include foods I never would have thought of putting together, which has opened up a whole new world of meals for me and my family.

"My energy level has also improved dramatically. After the birth of my son, I was constantly sleepy because of my thyroid disease, and being a new mom certainly didn't help either! On *Eat Carbs, Lose Weight,* I'm in a better mood and feel more energetic all the time.

"Best of all, I've had quite a few people tell me I looked great. My husband is constantly telling me that I look noticeably smaller, and the rest of my family and friends have all told me how good I look. Actually, my family and friends can't wait for the book to come out so they can try the diet, too. It feels wonderful! Without *Eat Carbs, Lose Weight,* I would still be struggling on every diet out there and not being successful. I will continue on the diet until I reach my goal weight loss of 80 pounds. On Denise's plan, I know I can do it."

Devan's advice: "Believe you can accomplish your weight-loss goals. Even if you don't see a lower number on the scale, you may be losing inches. Sometimes I would be a little depressed if I didn't see the scale move, but then I'd check my measurements and see I was actually losing more inches than pounds."

All of these extra calories add up. No matter whether they come from carbs, fat, or protein, extra calories do one and only one thing—they make themselves comfy in the fat cells in your thighs, hips, buns, and belly.

In addition to the hidden calories they were getting from processed foods, many low-fat dieters were overeating for another reason: They were hungry and deprived. Most of the carbs people consumed during the 1970s, '80s, and '90s were starchy, refined, and high in sugar. Such foods score high on something called the glycemic index, a ranking of carbohydrate foods based on how quickly the body breaks them down and converts them into blood sugar. Research shows that when humans eat foods high on the index, a sequence of hormonal changes takes place that causes them to overeat.

Because the body breaks down these foods quickly, too much sugar enters the blood-stream at too fast a rate. To bring blood sugar levels down, the pancreas responds by secreting high amounts of the hormone insulin. This hormone is responsible for shuttling blood sugar into hungry cells around your body, which burn the sugar for energy.

When the pancreas secretes too much insulin, however, the hormone clears blood sugar too quickly. Blood sugar levels then drop. You end up feeling hungry soon after eating. You'll also begin to crave the very foods—sweets—that caused the blood sugar roller-coaster ride in the first place.

In addition to spiking blood sugar, meals that contain all carbohydrate and no fat or protein will make you feel hungry for yet another reason. Fat and protein help to slow digestion and make you feel sated. Fat, in particular, helps to make food taste good.

You may have noticed this phenomenon yourself if you've ever eaten a plain bagel for breakfast. Although the bagel contains more than 400 calories—which should be plenty to power you through the morning—you probably felt hungry again just 1 or 2 hours later. You also may notice this if you've ever eaten refined white pasta with red sauce for dinner. If you dished up just one serving—which is *much* smaller than what most people typically put on their plates—you probably began rooting around in your cabinets for cookies and other sweet foods as soon as you finished washing the dishes (assuming you could even wait that long).

I hear about this problem all the time from my girlfriends and fans. They tell me that they hardly eat anything, yet they can't lose weight. When I ask them what they eat, I find out that they eat a slice of toast with jam for breakfast (if they eat breakfast at all) and survive on a salad with fat-free dressing at lunch. By midafternoon, they are ravenous and consequently dive into whatever fat-free snack they can find at the closest vending machine. Once they get home from work, they raid the refrigerator and lose all willpower, eating more calories in one meal than they should be eating all day long.

All of this said, you can eat the bread and pasta and other carbs you love—and still feel satisfied. You just need to eat the *right* carbs in the *right* amounts, balancing your carbohydrate consumption with your fat and protein consumption. The *Eat Carbs, Lose Weight* meal plan will teach you how to do just that.

WHY LOW-CARB DIETS DON'T WORK

People gained weight during the fat-phobic 1980s and 1990s for two reasons. They ate too many of the wrong types of carbs, and they consumed too many calories. It's that simple. They were out of balance.

Low-carb diets, however, are just as out of balance as the low-fat diets. As with the low-fat diets, low-carbohydrate diets do result in weight loss. They do work in the short term. They may not, however, work in the long term.

The longest study done on low-carb diets lasted only 1 year. In this study, participants lost roughly the same amount of weight on a low-carb diet as others who followed a low-fat diet. One year, however, doesn't provide enough time to test whether dieters can keep off the weight once they lose it. It's also not long enough to determine the possible adverse health effects of these diets.

Amy Campbell and I suspect that long-term studies will reveal that low-carb dieters tend to gain back more weight than they lost in the first place—just as low-fat dieters have done. Although it certainly wasn't a scientific study, I do have some evidence to back up our belief. When I asked more than 30 of my fans about their results from low-carb diets, they told me that they did lose weight at first but gained back all of it—and in some cases more—once they lost the motivation to stick with the diet. Many said they felt hungrier when they tried low-carb diets and that their cravings for carbs intensified dramatically. They also felt fatigued and experienced a dull headache during the time they were on the diet.

"When I tried the low-carb approach, I craved carbs to extremes, to the point of getting sick," one fan, Susie Fox, told me. Another fan, Colleen M. Barricklow, said, "It was easy for the first few days, and then it got harder. I found that once I started eating any carbs, all the weight came right back and then some."

To understand why they experienced such negative results, you need to understand how low-carb diets work. Low-carbohydrate diets probably result in weight loss by forcing your body to burn fat for energy. Your body prefers to burn carbohydrate—either from blood sugar or from the stored carbohydrate in your liver and muscles (called glycogen). When you reduce your carbohydrate consumption to almost nothing, however, your body quickly runs through its supplies of blood sugar and stored glycogen. It then turns to what it has left: fat and protein. Fat, of course, is what you want to burn. Protein is not.

When your body burns protein for energy, it raids the protein from your muscle tissue. Every pound of muscle in your body burns between 35 and 50 calories a day just to maintain itself. That's in addition to the countless additional calories your muscles burn when they power every move your body makes. When you lose muscle protein, you slow your metabolism. This sets you up for weight gain down the road—when you abandon your low-carb lifestyle.

If you could stick to eating low carb for the rest of your life, you might not regain the weight. Few people last this long, however. Studies show that about 40 percent of people cheat and eventually drop out of low-carb diets. By the way, that's roughly the same percentage of people who lose the motivation to stick with low-fat diets.

With longer-term studies, we also may find that these diets are anything but good for your health. When you force your body to burn fat in the absence of carbohydrate, your body cannot burn fat completely. This creates by-products called ketones. Normally, your body can clear these ketones from your blood, but when it burns fat too quickly, they can build up to dangerous levels. This may increase levels of uric acid in your blood, which raises your risk for gout and kidney stones.

Carbohydrates also house a number of healthful nutrients—such as fiber—not found in protein and fatty foods. Carbohydrate-rich foods such as fruits and vegetables contain numerous phytonutrients—not found in meat—that can help prevent many types of disease. When you cut carbs from your diet, you lose out on these important nutrients. Although more research is needed to be sure, many scientists believe studies will

Are Low-Carb Diets Good for Your Heart?

Perhaps in a health magazine or on the 6 o'clock news, you learned about research that found a positive relationship between low-carbohydrate diets and heart health. For example, one of these studies, completed at the University of Connecticut, found that a diet that derived only 10 percent of calories from carbs increased LDL cholesterol particle size, which makes these undesirable components less likely to clog your arteries. The low-carb diet also lowered triglycerides, a type of blood fat that raises risk for heart disease. Studies completed at Duke University and the University of Pennsylvania have produced similar findings.

Does this mean that low-carb diets are good for your heart? Not necessarily. Any diet that results in weight loss—low fat, low carb, or something else—is good for your heart, at least in the short term. That's because *weight loss* itself is good for the heart. Indeed, when 650 obese patients underwent gastric banding surgery, they improved their blood sugar and blood cholesterol levels—even though they didn't change their diets.

Until longer-term studies are completed, it's hard to predict the long-term effects of low-carb diets on heart health. Researchers have shown time and time again that a diet rich in fiber, fruits, vegetables, whole grains, and legumes (all carbohydrate foods) reduces the risk for not only heart disease but also stroke, diabetes, and cancer. In time, I'm confident that we will find out that omitting these foods from your diet is not wise.

eventually show that low-carb diets—because they lack these important nutrients—raise the risk for heart disease and cancer.

Finally, and possibly most important, low-carb diets lower your quality of life. As you will learn in chapter 2, your body and brain prefer to burn carbs for energy. Cut out the carbs and you feel tired, muddled, and grumpy. Carbs also taste so good. And that's very important! Life's too short to forgo the foods you love.

THE TRUE SOURCE OF THE PROBLEM

Rather than eliminate carbs from the menu, most Americans simply need to eat less. Several studies now show that meal portions—both those served at restaurants and those dished up at home—have increased during the past 20 years.

As with most other animals, when we humans see food, we tend to eat it—even if we're not hungry. We're no different from the family dog that binges on an entire sheet of birthday cake when you're out of the room. The dog slurps up the cake as fast as possible for as long as possible and doesn't stop until either you catch him in the act or he's licked up every single crumb. He may certainly feel sick later on, but he doesn't learn from his miscalculation.

Humans are smarter than dogs in many respects; however, several studies show we may possess the same intelligence when it comes to eating. For example, researchers at Pennsylvania State University have tested how humans respond to different-sized meals. In one study, researchers observed the eating habits of customers at a restaurant. Customers who were served larger portions of pasta ate nearly all of the food on their plates—and 172 calories more than customers served smaller portions. Yet both sets of customers later rated their satisfaction after their meals similarly. The excess calories didn't make customers feel any more satisfied.

In another study completed at Penn State, researchers fed participants different-sized lunches over a period of weeks. Small portions or large, participants tended to eat everything on their plates—but felt just as satisfied after eating a smaller portion as after a larger one.

These regular episodes of overeating have expanded our waistlines, which has made it harder to lose weight. As you gain weight, your body fails to process blood sugar efficiently. The hormone insulin usually acts like a key to unlock hungry body cells and escort sugar inside where it can be burned for energy. As you gain weight, however, your cells fail to recognize insulin.

When your cells respond poorly to insulin, your pancreas must secrete more and more insulin to help shuttle sugar into cells. Called insulin resistance, this can become a vicious cycle that can eventually lead to diabetes. Because your insulin isn't working as well as it should, blood sugar levels and insulin levels remain chronically high. You feel hungry, you crave the very foods you're trying not to eat, and you gain weight.

In a study of 465 people, researchers from Stanford University School of Medicine in California examined the relationship among body fat, blood sugar levels, and insulin levels. They asked each participant to eat 75 grams of sugar. Those who had the most body fat were more likely to be insulin resistant and have higher levels of the bad LDL

Size Matters: As Portions Grow Larger, So Do We

Studies completed at the University of North Carolina and the U.S. Department of Agriculture found that the following foods increased in serving size during the past 20 years.

Food	Number of Calories Each Portion Size Increased
Orange juice	15
Fruit drinks	30
Wine	30
Soft drinks	49
French fries	68
Salty snacks	93
Beer	96
Hamburgers	97
Mexican food	133

"I Ate Carbs and Lost Weight!"

Name: Megan Gjovig

Age: 20

Town: Nashville, Tennessee

Weight Lost: 5 pounds in 4 weeks

Other Accomplishments: Lost 13¼ inches and has been sticking with the plan to take her weight loss even further

"Like so many women, my diet was reasonably good and I exercised now and then, but I wasn't really doing either efficiently. As a result, I became 10 to 15 pounds overweight.

"*Eat Carbs, Lose Weight* was the first formal diet I've ever been on. In the past, I would cut back on various foods or integrate new nutrition tips I'd hear about, but this was the first time I did a specific diet for a specific amount of time . . . and it worked!

"I am a true believer in balanced nutrition, which is why *Eat Carbs, Lose Weight* was so attractive to me. I hate cutting foods out of my diet—and this diet still allowed me to eat a variety of tasty foods. This diet was a deliberate version of what I was trying to do—it gave me the guidance I needed.

"Specifically, I feel that a combination of proteins and carbohydrates is important, and the recipes that were part of *Eat Carbs, Lose Weight* incorporated a good balance of both.

"I am very pleased with the 13¼ inches I lost on my body—so pleased that I have been sticking with the plan to take my body shrinking even further. My personal trainer commented on the inches I lost even before we remeasured. He said he noticed that my legs got smaller. My family also noticed the change, which was motivating!"

Megan's advice: "Stay the course, and it will pay off. Once you've finished your initial 28 days, take the healthful principles of the diet and adapt them to your lifestyle. It is an easy plan to keep up."

cholesterol. Poor blood sugar control was also linked to higher triglycerides, a type of blood fat that raises your risk for heart disease.

The *Eat Carbs, Lose Weight* plan will help you to turn this vicious cycle around. Even if you already have insulin resistance or diabetes, you can lose weight and improve your body's sensitivity to insulin. Let's take a closer look at how the diet works.

HOW TO EAT YOUR CARBS—AND LOSE WEIGHT, TOO

Neither Amy nor I believe 80 or 90 percent of your diet should consist of carbs—or protein or fat, for that matter. We believe in balance. The meal plan in this book provides a moderate breakdown of carbs, protein, and fat. With our approach, you'll consume roughly 50 percent of your calories from carbs. This amount will help you to include enough fat and protein in your diet to slow digestion, feel satisfied after every meal, and keep blood sugar levels stable.

This breakdown is what Amy recommends to her patients with diabetes. That's right, even people with blood sugar problems can eat carbs—up to 50 percent of their total calories—and still keep blood sugar levels in check.

Consider these facts:

❖ A study with roughly the same carb-protein-fat breakdown as ours was completed in Edinburgh, Scotland, and published recently in the *International Journal of Food Sciences and Nutrition*. In this study, researchers fed 76 men who classified themselves as emotional eaters a diet that contained 54 percent carbs, 20 percent protein, and 26 percent fat. After 12 weeks, the men not only lost weight but also experienced fewer cravings and felt better about sugar-containing foods—and about life in general.

❖ A study completed at the University of Guelph in Ontario compared a low-fat diet (17 percent of calories from fat) with a low-carbohydrate diet (15 percent of calories from carbs). Both groups lost the same amount of weight on the scale, but the low-carb group lost more muscle mass, whereas the low-fat group lost more fat. As I've mentioned, this is important because your muscle mass is the one aspect of your metabolism that's under your control. Each pound of muscle burns between 35 and 50 calories a day to maintain itself. Less muscle equals a slower metabolism, which sets you up for future weight gain.

In addition to providing the best balance of carbohydrates, protein, and fat for weight loss, the *Eat Carbs, Lose Weight* approach will help you shed fat in a few other important ways. First, and most important, the meals included in your meal plan are all low in something called glycemic load. In 1981, the *American Journal of Clinical Nutrition* released the glycemic index (GI), a ranking of how quickly the body breaks down certain foods and converts them into blood sugar. The index rates hundreds of foods on a scale from 0 to 100. Foods that break down quickly and enter the bloodstream the fastest have the highest index ratings (more than 70), whereas foods that break down and enter the bloodstream the slowest have the lowest ratings (less than 55).

Foods high on the index tend to result in less satiety and more calorie consumption than foods lower on the index. A recent study from Children's Hospital in Boston found that simply switching from a high-GI diet to a low one—without necessarily lowering the amount of carbohydrate in the diet—helped obese teenagers shed fat. This type of diet allows you to have your carbs and lose weight, too because you will feel more satisfied for a longer period of time, so you won't be headed back to the pantry for another snack fix!

The glycemic load (GL) takes the glycemic index a step further, making it a bit more useful to you. For example, some foods—such as carrots, watermelon, and pumpkin—rate high on the index but don't necessarily result in sky-high blood sugar. These foods may hit your bloodstream quickly, but they don't contain enough carbohydrate calories to greatly affect blood sugar levels.

That's where glycemic load comes in. Glycemic load is measured in "glycemic units," the result of a simple mathematical computation. (We'll include it here, but don't worry—you'll *never* have to do any math on this plan. We've done all the calculations for you.)

To calculate the glycemic load of a particular food, you multiply that food's glycemic index by the number of grams of carbohydrate in a serving, then divide by 100. For example, a teaspoon of jam has a glycemic load of 2.5:

$$
\begin{array}{rl}
51 & \text{(the glycemic index of jam)} \\
\times \quad 5 & \text{(the grams of carbohydrate in 1 teaspoon of jam)} \\
\div \quad 100 & \\
\hline
= \quad 2.5 & \text{(the glycemic load)}
\end{array}
$$

Ideally, you want your *total* glycemic load (the sum of each portion of your food's glycemic load added all together) to be below 80 for the day. Most people consume a diet with a daily GL of closer to 100. The recipes and meals included in the *Eat Carbs, Lose Weight* meal plans are all low in glycemic load.

Each meal you eat on the *Eat Carbs, Lose Weight* plan is also rich in fiber, a nutrient that is found *only* in carbohydrate foods. (This is another reason why carbs are so essential!) Fiber helps suppress the appetite by delaying stomach emptying after you eat. It also slows the rate at which the food you eat is absorbed into your bloodstream. This helps to keep blood sugar levels stable, controlling hunger and keeping energy levels high. Various studies have linked consumption of fiber to a lower body mass index (BMI), a relationship of weight to height. The lower the BMI, the thinner the person.

Bottom line: To stick to any diet long term, you must enjoy it. Your diet must be palatable. It actually *should* taste delicious. If you love carbs, how can you give them up? The answer is that you shouldn't. No one needs to sacrifice so much to lose weight!

YOUR FUTURE SUCCESS

The *Eat Carbs, Lose Weight* plan is designed to help you to lose up to 2 pounds of fat a week. Each day, you will consume about 1,300 calories spread out over three meals and two snacks. During each meal, you will eat balanced portions of carbohydrates, protein, and fat. You will consume the best carbs—those that are packed with nutrients and fiber and come straight from Mother Nature. All together: You'll lose weight without feeling hungry or deprived.

As you lose weight, you'll firm up and boost your metabolism with my Daily Dozen routine. This series of 12 exercises in chapter 5 will help you to sculpt the muscle you need to increase your metabolism. This entire routine takes just 12 minutes. It's the easiest and most efficient exercise routine I've ever designed. I'm confident that you will love it . . . and do it! It's your "minimum daily requirement."

In addition to looking better, you will also feel better. The *Eat Carbs, Lose Weight* plan will do more than help you shed fat. It will finally, once and for all, put you in control of your eating. By eating the right foods in the right proportions, you will rein in emotional eating, reduce your cravings, and put an end to overeating. You'll form a truce with the most tempting of foods and no longer feel guilty about what you eat.

You'll also improve your health. As you lose weight, your body will process blood sugar more efficiently, and you'll be less likely to have sugar and insulin problems. A review of numerous studies done at the University of Toronto concluded that the best diet for improving health was one that was rich in monounsaturated fats, fiber, and low-GI foods. That's exactly what the *Eat Carbs, Lose Weight* plan recommends.

The *Eat Carbs, Lose Weight* plan includes the best foods nature has to offer. On this plan, you can expect to lower your blood sugar, triglycerides, and blood pressure within just 1 to 2 weeks. Your blood cholesterol will begin to drop after 3 weeks.

Better health. More savory meals. More energy. Better moods. A slimmer body. What are you waiting for? Turn to chapter 2 to discover the many varied reasons why you can finally say yes to carbs.

THE RETURN OF CARBS

Why you can—and should—put carbs back on your plate

Wherever I go, I hear from people who have tried to give up carbs. They complain they are too tired to exercise. They tell me they can't concentrate at work. Some are irritable. Others can't sleep well at night. Still others say they find themselves bingeing on sugary carbohydrate foods like brownies.

Although many ask me for tips on finding the willpower to stick with their diets, I usually offer the following advice. "Willpower is not your problem," I say. "Your diet is your problem." In my opinion, these people have tons of willpower. Anyone who can stop eating her favorite foods and put up with side effects such as fatigue and insomnia for *any* length of time has plenty of willpower. Trying to stick to a low-carb diet goes against human nature. You see, we humans are genetically programmed to enjoy carbohydrates.

Whether it's the crunch of popcorn or the sweet taste of fruit, carbohydrate foods make our mouths water. When we eat these foods, we feel good. Plus, you'll soon learn, carbohydrate foods actually stimulate brain chemicals that boost mood, rewarding us for eating them.

This dates back to our hunting and gathering days. Our early ancestors consumed a balanced diet that included carbohydrates from the fruit and nuts they gathered and proteins and fats from the wild animals they hunted. During those early years, humans learned to enjoy the sweet tastes of berries and other carbs because these foods provided the energy and nutrition they needed to thrive.

Today, berries and other carbohydrate foods continue to help us stay healthy. I'm no exception. Most days, I have cereal with fat-free milk and berries for breakfast. Starting the day with the sweet taste of fruit has helped me to feel satisfied and it's balanced. I'm less likely to overeat during the day and more likely to control my weight.

Many studies bear this out. In a study completed by the U.S. Department of Agriculture, researchers looked at the eating habits and body sizes of more than 10,000 adults. This study, published in the *Journal of the American College of Nutrition*, found that adults who consumed about 55 percent of their calories from carbohydrates (roughly the amount of carbs included in the *Eat Carbs, Lose Weight* meal plan) were more likely to remain at a healthy weight than adults who ate less carbohydrate.

Why You Should Honor Your Sweet Tooth

When a sweet tooth begs to be satisfied, many people turn to cake, cookies, chocolate, and other foods made from refined sugar and flour. Unlike the wholesome and nutrition-packed berries and other fruit that our early ancestors consumed, these refined carbohydrates offer empty calories. That doesn't, however, make them worthless.

It's true that eating too many of these refined carbs and too few of the wholesome carbs from Mother Earth can indeed set you up for weight gain. You need not, however, give up chocolate and your other favorite foods in order to lose weight. In fact, doing so will only increase your cravings for these very foods, reducing your chances of success. Rather than trying to muster the willpower needed to shun your favorite foods, you need only strike a careful balance between wholesome natural carbs and refined ones. The *Eat Carbs, Lose Weight* meal plan does just that. I love to nibble on frozen pineapple chunks or frozen mango pieces—a great healthy dessert or treat!

Carbs offer so many benefits in addition to weight loss that it's hard for me to believe that anyone would come up with a diet that recommends against eating them. I think of veggies, whole-grain bread, fresh fruit, and many other high-carbohydrate foods as essential. I hope that after reading this chapter, you will feel the same. (You'll also learn more about the best types of carbohydrates for weight loss in chapter 4.)

WHAT ARE CARBS?

To understand why carbs are so good for you, you must first understand what they are. While protein mainly comes from animal products such as eggs and meat, carbohydrates are found in plant foods such as legumes, fruits, vegetables, and grains. Let's not forget the cocoa plant and sugarcane. Without them, we wouldn't have some of our tastiest foods.

Of course, not all high-carbohydrate foods resemble their original source. Bread and crackers, for example, are made from wheat and other grains. Potato chips come from potatoes. Even cake comes from plant foods: sugarcane and the wheat that made the flour.

There are four main types of carbs. They include:

1. Simple sugars. Found in honey (glucose), table sugar (sucrose), fruit (fructose), and milk (lactose), these types contain just one or two units of sugar per molecule. Because they are so small, your intestine can absorb them directly into your bloodstream without first breaking them down into smaller units. Many years ago, food scientists warned us to stay away from simple sugars and to opt for more complex carbohydrates (such as starch and fiber) instead. The reasoning was that, because the body didn't have to break down simple sugars before absorbing them into the bloodstream, these sugars could cause large swings in blood sugar, resulting in fatigue and overeating. This, however, isn't necessarily the case, as you will learn in chapter 4.

2. Fiber. Fiber (and starch, below) is considered "complex" because it contains three or more chains of sugar units per molecule. Once called roughage or bulk, fiber gained attention back in the 1960s when the high-fiber diets of rural people living in nonindustrialized nations were linked to a lower incidence of heart disease. Digestive enzymes cannot break fiber down into simple sugars, so it passes through your gut largely undigested. This offers many benefits, including better colon health, reduced risk for heart disease, and a lower appetite.

3. Starch. Similar in chemical structure to fiber, starch is a type of sugar found in potatoes, rice, and many other plant foods. Plants, especially root vegetables and grains, store sugar in the form of starch. Although low-carb diets would have you believe that all starch is bad, this again isn't necessarily true. Some types of starches, called resistant starch, act like fiber in the gut. They resist digestion, passing through the intestine intact, especially when eaten raw.

4. Oligosaccharides. They're more complex than simple sugars and less complex than starch and fiber. Although there are many types of oligosaccharides, two in particular—raffinose and stachyose—will greatly aid your weight-loss efforts. Found in beans and other legumes, these carbs act like fiber in the gut. They resist digestion, traveling through the gut largely intact. This helps to stabilize blood sugar, reduce appetite, and maintain your energy levels.

Digestive enzymes in your intestine break down most of the carbs you eat into glucose, a single-sugar molecule that can be absorbed through your intestinal wall and into your bloodstream. Glucose floats around in your bloodstream until hungry cells throughout your body burn it for energy. This is why carbs are so important. They are your body's primary energy source. Carbs power nearly every action in the body, from muscle movements to brain activity. They help maintain your bodily organs and nerve cells. You need carbs to survive!

Your body tries to keep the amount of glucose in your blood at a consistent level. When blood glucose levels drop too low, your body sends out hormones that make you feel hungry. When blood glucose levels are too high, it sends out other hormones to bring blood glucose levels down by storing those carbs as fat and glycogen.

The hormone insulin is one of many hormones that regulate the flow of sugar to and from your blood. As blood glucose rises, cells in your pancreas sense this rise and send out more insulin to bring it down. If there are not enough hungry cells to soak up the glucose and burn it, insulin and other hormones signal your body to convert the excess into glycogen and store it in your muscles and liver. Your muscles and liver can house only about three-quarters of a pound of glycogen, so if you really overwhelm your

The Science of Carbohydrates

Sugar molecules form the building blocks of all carbs and are classified according to how many units combine to form one sugar molecule. For example, a monosaccharide— a fancy word that simply means "one sugar"—has just one sugar unit. Monosaccharides are considered simple sugars. When two of them combine, they form another type of simple sugar called a disaccharide, which literally means "two sugars." For example, table sugar is a combination of the monosaccharides glucose and fructose. Oligosaccharides are a combination of three to nine sugar units per molecule, and polysaccharides contain more than 10 units per molecule.

Here's an overview of different types of carbohydrates and which foods contain them.

Carbohydrate	Specific Types	Foods That Contain This Type of Carbohydrate
Sugar	Fructose	Fruit
	Galactose	Honey
	Glucose	Milk
	Lactose	Table sugar
	Sucrose	
Oligosaccharides	Maltodextrins	Artichokes
	Raffinose	Beans
	Stachyose	Onions
		Soy products
Polysaccharides (starch and fiber)	Cellulose, hemicelluloses	Bread
	Hydrocolloids	Fruit
	Pectin	Rice

bloodstream with glucose and your liver and muscles are already full, the excess is converted into fat and stored in your fat cells.

HOW CARBS PROMOTE WEIGHT LOSS

Fiber and other nondigestible carbohydrates work wonderful weight-loss magic. Think of these carbs as negative calories. As fiber and other nondigestible carbs pass through your intestine undigested, they bring other nutrients—often fat—along for the ride. This prevents your intestine from breaking down and absorbing some of the fat and cholesterol from the food you eat. How do scientists know this? They followed some people into the bathroom!

Researchers in the lab examined the stool of volunteers after they consumed meals with differing amounts of fiber. The more fiber the participants ate, the more fat the researchers found in their stools.

Fiber and other nondigestible carbs are bulky and tend to slow digestion, which, in turn, eases the absorption of glucose into the bloodstream. When glucose enters the bloodstream more slowly, cells are better able to burn it for energy. End result: Your body will burn more sugar and store less of it as fat.

Because glucose moves into your bloodstream at a leisurely pace, blood glucose and insulin levels also remain stable. High levels of insulin signal you to feel hungry—particularly for high-calorie carbs. Consistent insulin levels, on the other hand, help to drive down hunger and reduce the cravings that can lead to bingeing.

Because fiber and other nondigestible carbs delay stomach emptying, the body processes a fiber-rich meal more slowly. This makes you feel full sooner (so you stop eating earlier). Foods that are high in fiber also tend to be less "energy dense," which means they are low in calories per volume. They are also bulky and filling. When you eat foods high in fiber, you feel full faster, making you less likely to overeat.

Research completed at Tufts University in Boston found that consuming 14 more grams of fiber in a day results in an automatic 10 percent decrease in calorie consump-

"I Ate Carbs and Lost Weight!"

Name: Kaci Sohrt
Age: 29
Town: Austin, Texas
Weight Loss: 12½ pounds in 4 weeks
Accomplishments: Lost a total of 14 inches off her body

"Like so many women, I gained weight by accident. As my schedule got tighter, so did my pants. As a full-time law student with a part-time job, I started skipping exercise, eating on the run, and grabbing a muffin at school for breakfast and fast food for lunch. I also started dating a new guy (now my fiancé), which was wonderful but also led to a lot of high-calorie dinners out. All that combined with steroid shots I started taking to deal with pain from a previous surgery led me to gain weight.

"After having tried the diet drug Calotren (which just led to more weight gain!), Weight Watchers, and Slim-Fast without success, I was frustrated. I was intrigued by *Eat Carbs, Lose Weight* because I trust Denise and her nutrition advice, and the plan just seemed to make more sense to me than a lot of other diets out there that leave out entire food groups. Since I had just gotten engaged and wanted to slim down for my wedding, Denise and her program came along at the perfect time!

"The variety of foods and delicious recipes in *Eat Carbs, Lose Weight* have made it easy for me to stick to, and I've loved being able to eat snacks during the day. I noticed my cravings for 'bad' foods disappeared, especially after I started to see results.

"And best of all, my fiancé loves the recipes, too. It was nice for both of us to get out of our rut and try new foods. I even made a few of the recipes when my family came to visit, and they raved about them even though they were part of a 'diet' plan.

"I am thrilled with the 12½ pounds and 14 inches I lost. My fiancé thinks I look like I lost 20 pounds. I am really encouraged and plan to maintain the program together with a regular exercise routine. Thanks, Denise!"

Kaci's advice: "Planning is everything. Plan a week at a time based on your personal schedule, including room for leftovers and unavoidable eating out. Buy frozen fruits and vegetables when you can—they're cleaned and ready to go, and they keep longer for when you need only a small amount of a recipe. If you find you're still hungry, make a plain salad with fat-free Italian dressing."

tion. So if you usually consume 2,000 calories a day, adding this much fiber to your daily menu will cause you to eat 200 fewer calories simply because you don't feel as hungry! If you are like most Americans, you probably consume fewer than 15 grams of fiber a day. The *Eat Carbs, Lose Weight* meal plans include 20 to 35 grams of fiber a day, which will help you to feel more satisfied on fewer calories.

Possibly *because* it helps you to feel more full on less food, fiber can help accelerate weight loss. In research completed at Tufts University, a low-fat, high-fiber diet resulted in three times more weight loss than a low-fat, low-fiber diet. That's incredible!

Don't forget, carbohydrate foods are the only foods on the planet that house fiber and other nondigestible carbs. When you go on a low-carb diet, you shortchange your body of these important weight-loss benefits.

ADDITIONAL BENEFITS OF CARBS

Besides adding wonderful tastes and textures to so many savory foods, carbs provide your body with energy. Carbohydrates break down into the sugar that powers your muscle movements, brain activity, and many other cell interactions. Your body also uses carbs to build and maintain bodily organs and nerve cells.

When eaten as part of a balanced diet, carbs have many wonderful benefits. They include the following.

Improved Mood

Carbohydrates help boost mood in many ways, but possibly the most important is by their effect on the brain chemical serotonin. Your brain houses a number of substances called neurotransmitters, chemical messengers that relay important information from one neuron (or brain cell) to another. Levels of these messengers influence many of your body's functions, including your mood, appetite, thoughts, and even behavior.

One of these messengers, serotonin, promotes feelings of joy, optimism, and calm. When serotonin levels are optimal, you sleep better, feel better, and think better. You have fewer cravings and are less likely to overeat. On the other hand, when levels of this neurotransmitter drop too low, you feel depressed and irritable, may crave sugary foods, and are more likely to overeat, particularly when you are under stress.

So it only makes good sense that you'd want to keep levels of this important brain chemical optimal. Yet, low-carb diets do the opposite.

At the Massachusetts Institute of Technology, research scientists Judith and Richard Wurtman have spent much of their careers studying the effects of carbohydrates, proteins, and fats on mood. After conducting many studies spanning many years on mice and on humans, they've concluded that carbohydrates are particularly important for optimal mood. In fact, Judith Wurtman refers to the depression, anger, and tension that tend to surface when participants try low-carb diets as "the Atkins attitude."

In studies they've conducted on rats, the Wurtmans have discovered that dietary carbohydrates help keep serotonin levels optimal. When researchers fed rats a low-carb diet, levels of this mood-boosting brain chemical dropped. The rats also overate their chow. Another study, completed in the Netherlands, found a high protein, low-carb diet increased levels of perceived stress and fatigue in stress-prone participants. Additional research has found that most dieters feel depressed after about 2 weeks on a low-carb diet, around the time this brain chemical drops due to a decrease in carbohydrate consumption.

Various amino acids from your food increase the production of different types of brain chemicals. The brain uses one amino acid in particular, tryptophan, to manufacture serotonin. Although amino acids come from protein foods, the carbohydrate you eat can influence whether optimal amounts of tryptophan cross into your brain.

When you eat high-carbohydrate foods, your blood insulin levels rise. Insulin directs many amino acids into cells throughout your body. This suppresses blood levels of the amino acids that compete with tryptophan for entrance into the brain. It's similar to waiting in line to pass through customs after an international flight. You can't go home until you pass a gatekeeper—in this case, the customs agent. Everyone in the room wants to get past the gatekeeper as quickly as possible. Some people get through quickly, whereas others must open their luggage, answer numerous questions, and have their passports examined more closely. You know you'll feel better once you get to the other side and out of the airport, but you must compete with many other passengers to get there.

Carbohydrates put tryptophan in the fast line and clear out the room, sending the competing amino acids elsewhere. This allows tryptophan to easily and quickly pass through customs (the blood-brain barrier) and enter the brain, causing neurons to make more serotonin.

When you eat too much protein and too little carbohydrate, however, you risk raising the levels of other neurotransmitters too high. Amino acids in protein foods such as fish increase amounts of the amino acid tyrosine in the brain, which the brain uses to manufacture neurotransmitters such as norepinephrine. When in normal amounts, these brain chemicals make you feel energetic and alert. But when they are too high, you feel agitated and anxious, as if you just drank too much coffee.

In addition to boosting serotonin, carbohydrate influences your mood in a few other important ways. Many carbohydrate foods—especially fortified breakfast cereal and dark leafy greens—are rich in folate. Deficiencies in this vitamin have been linked to depression. This vitamin is found predominantly in carbohydrate foods, so when you go on a low-carb diet, you may become deficient in folate.

Any food you find delicious, whether it's whole-grain bread or chocolate, will boost levels of the brain chemical dopamine, another feel-good neurotransmitter that increases feelings of pleasure. This is one reason why it's important to include small amounts of some of your most delectable foods in your weight-loss plan—even if they are full of sugar. These foods will help occasionally boost this brain chemical, making you feel good on a regular basis. See—maybe you really do owe yourself that cookie!

Finally, low blood glucose levels can also make you feel irritable and moody. You must eat carbs, especially those low on the glycemic index, to keep blood sugar levels optimal.

Fewer Cravings

For the same reasons carbohydrates boost mood, they also help curb your cravings. When you stop eating carbohydrate, the brain stops regulating serotonin and sends out signals that encourage you to eat carbohydrates. If you eat protein instead, you'll get grumpy, irritable, or restless—and your cravings for carbs will get even stronger.

Researchers in New Zealand highlighted the importance of carbs and cravings with the following experiment. They offered nine women three different types of meals on three separate days. The women had previously reported feeling intense cravings for specific foods. The meals were either high in protein, high in carbs, or a balanced mix of protein and carbs. After consuming the protein-rich meal—and not the high-carbohydrate or balanced meal—the women craved sweet carbohydrate foods. Later in the day, participants binged on foods that were high in sugar and fat. Participants also reported feeling depressed and moody after eating the high-protein meal.

In another study, completed at MIT, researchers asked women with premenstrual syndrome to consume a carbohydrate-rich beverage during the time of their cycle when they were most likely to feel mood swings and crave carbs. After they drank the beverage, their cravings for carbs decreased and they felt less depressed, angry, and confused.

Better Digestion

While better digestion may not be the most glamorous benefit, it is very important to many facets of optimum health and efficient weight loss. You see, fiber—both insoluble and soluble—helps to keep you regular. Insoluble fiber, which makes up the walls of plant cells, passes through your intestine intact. Though mashed, it remains stiff and adds bulk to your feces. This stimulates your intestines, causing muscles along the walls of your intestines to initiate the wavelike motion called peristalsis that pushes stool through the intestine. Soluble fiber, on the other hand, absorbs water during its trip through your intestine. Once in the colon, this fiber becomes gel-like, softening your stool and making it easier to pass.

Normally, it takes anywhere from 12 to 36 hours for food to pass from your stomach through your intestines. This is the ideal amount of time for this trip. When you eat less fiber, however, the passage of food slows. When food sits in your intestines too long, the bacteria in your gut ferment it for too long a period of time, causing gas, indigestion, and bloating. Another consequence: Your stool dries out, which results in constipation and uncomfortable elimination.

A faster transit time through the colon offers another benefit: a reduced incidence of colon cancer. When stool moves through your colon more quickly, it more quickly whisks carcinogens out of your body.

Softer, easier-to-pass stools can also prevent a host of other problems, from hemorrhoids to anal fissures to a disease called diverticulosis (when the intestinal wall becomes inflamed or infected). In a study published in the *American Journal of Clinical Nutrition*, men who ate high-fiber diets reduced their risk of developing diverticulosis by 50 percent compared with men who consumed low-fiber diets.

Fiber also helps to promote the growth of beneficial intestinal bacteria, such as Lactobacillus and Bifidus. These bacteria help break down food and create an acidic environment that keeps harmful bacteria in check. These bacteria also create nutrients that your body needs. For example, bacteria convert the folate you eat into folic acid. They also create the B vitamin biotin (important for blood sugar control), vitamin B_{12} (important in heart disease prevention), and vitamin K (important for strong bones). When you don't eat enough fiber, harmful bacteria can overwhelm the beneficial bacteria in your gut, which can cause diarrhea.

Where to Find Fiber

Many foods provide both insoluble and soluble fiber, whereas others contain predominantly one type over another. Both kinds are important, because they perform different functions in the body. Insoluble fiber primarily keeps your digestive tract running smoothly, whereas soluble fiber slows digestion, promotes feelings of fullness, reduces blood cholesterol, and stabilizes blood sugar levels.

Foods rich in insoluble fiber: apples, artichokes, beans, beets, berries, brussels sprouts, cabbage, carrots, cauliflower, corn, grapes, nuts, pears, prunes, turnips, whole-grain foods

Foods rich in soluble fiber: apples, barley, beans, broccoli, carrots, citrus fruit, flaxseeds, oats, pears, peas, prunes, rice, soy products, spinach, yams

More Alertness and Improved Memory

You need carbs to fuel your muscles and brain. Your brain in particular can burn *only* glucose—and not fat—for energy. Research shows that it needs a *minimum* of 130 grams of carbohydrates a day to function. (Most low-carb diets recommend you eat fewer than 40 grams a day.) When you skimp on carbs and your blood glucose levels remain chronically low, you'll begin to feel muddled, have trouble concentrating, and perhaps even notice poor memory recall. Indeed, research completed by the U.S. Army has shown that soldiers competing in intense training must consume carbs in order to function with a high level of mental alertness.

Elsewhere, in one study, researchers asked senior citizens to drink one of three beverages first thing in the morning: a protein beverage, a fatty beverage, or a high-carbohydrate beverage. When the seniors drank the carbohydrate beverage, they performed better on various memory tests an hour later. Indeed, the carbs/concentration link may be most important first thing in the morning, as many studies show schoolchildren who eat breakfast tend to perform better in school than children who skip breakfast. In one study, children who ate a carbohydrate-rich breakfast (Cheerios or shredded wheat) had improved attention and memory recall compared with children who didn't eat breakfast.

Increased Energy

Although your muscles *can* burn fat and even protein for fuel, they prefer to burn carbs, either from the glycogen stored in your muscles or liver or from the glucose in your blood. When you skimp on carbs, however, glycogen and blood glucose levels run low, and your muscles must switch to burning fat and protein. They end up cannibalizing themselves, making themselves weaker and slowing your metabolism. This not only slows your metabolism but can also make you feel fatigued in the long term as your muscles become weaker.

Remember that your body wants to keep blood glucose at a consistent level. When

"I Ate Carbs and Lost Weight!"

Name: Mary Rita Muldoon

Age: 43

Town: Los Angeles, California

Weight Lost: 7 pounds in 4 weeks

Other Accomplishments: Lost 4½ inches and felt liberated by the flexibility of the meal plans

"Having been a thin person most of my life, I was used to being able to eat what I wanted without ever worrying about calories, fats, or portions. But after I reached age 35, things changed and the weight slowly crept on. I tried a number of different diets, including Atkins and the blood type diet, but I had no luck. On Atkins, I just seemed to gain *more* weight. . . .

"Then one day it dawned on me: When I was thinner, I was eating plenty of carbs mixed with healthy proteins. I'm not a snacker—I just love to eat lots of 'good' foods. So maybe what I needed was to find a diet that incorporated these elements. *Eat Carbs, Lose Weight* turned out to be perfect for me—it was designed more for my metabolism with portion-controlled carbohydrates.

"On the diet, I felt like I was eating regularly and I never felt hungry. I no longer had specific rules for carbs, fats, and so forth. It was liberating to be able to eat well-balanced, portion-controlled meals just like normal people do. I had plenty of energy, and I was easily able to complete my 30 minutes of exercise, three or four times a week.

"After 28 days, I lost 7 pounds and 4½ inches. I am encouraged because the weight loss seems sustainable. A few people have asked me if I lost weight, but I think I've noticed the difference more than anyone. My clothes fit much better, and best of all, I have the energy and enthusiasm to keep going. I plan to continue on the diet until I reach my goal weight."

Mary Rita's advice: "Always be prepared with alternatives because life regularly throws you curveballs that can divert you from your goals. When I ate in restaurants on the diet, I tried to choose something similar to one of the recipes. At work, I stocked myself with healthful snacks and mini-meals just in case a meeting lasted through lunch and I didn't get a chance to eat."

levels drop too low, levels of a number of hormones rise to slow your metabolism (causing cells to burn less sugar) and slow your movements by making you feel tired. I competed as a gymnast through college, and I remember my coach telling us over and over again about the importance of carbohydrates for energy. He definitely was onto something, as numerous studies show that diets low in carbohydrate reduce athletic performance. In one study completed at the University of Birmingham in Edgbaston in the United Kingdom, researchers put runners on two different diets: one high in carbs and one low in carbs. When the runners consumed a low-carbohydrate diet, they felt more fatigued and reported feeling moody.

Researchers at the University Medical School in Aberdeen, Scotland, suspect a low-carb diet may make you feel fatigued for yet another reason. When your body switches to burning fat in the absence of carbohydrate, it creates by-products called ketones. As these build up in your blood, they may also make you feel tired.

Carbs are also the main fuel for exercise, especially high-intensity exercise. You must consume carbs to keep the glycogen stores in your muscles full—so your muscles can burn those stores when you move. When they are well stocked, you feel more energetic during your aerobics or power walking sessions.

Improved Health

Many carbohydrate foods are rich sources of vitamins, minerals, and substances called phytonutrients, which are chemicals found only in plants. Although we don't currently have a daily recommended amount of certain phytonutrients to eat each day, that does not make them any less important than vitamins and minerals. Plants make many of these chemicals in order to help themselves resist disease. When we eat them, they help us resist disease as well. Below, you'll find some examples of how phytonutrients help fend off all sorts of diseases, from cancer to cataracts.

⋄ **Lycopene.** The nutrient that lends tomatoes and ruby red grapefruit their red tint helps prevent the unhealthy LDL cholesterol from building up along artery walls. It also has been shown to reduce some types of cancer.

⬧ **Lutein and zeaxanthin.** Found in spinach, collards, and other dark leafy greens, these nutrients help reduce eye disease such as cataracts and macular degeneration.

⬧ **Bioflavonoids.** Found in citrus fruits such as lemons and oranges or other fruits such as apricots and cantaloupe, these phytonutrients help prevent cancer, heart disease, and diabetes.

⬧ **Indoles.** Found in cruciferous vegetables such as cauliflower, indoles help fight heart disease and cancer.

⬧ **Thioallyls.** Found in garlic and onions, these phytonutrients help lower blood cholesterol and prevent the formation of blood clots.

In addition to these important nutrients, carbohydrate foods are the only foods on the planet that supply fiber. The soluble fiber found in bran, oats, and barley helps lower cholesterol. Researchers at Harvard who studied the diets of thousands of women concluded that a diet that includes 25 grams of fiber a day reduces heart attack risk by 40 percent. Other research shows that adults who consume more fiber tend to have lower cholesterol levels and blood pressure. They are also less likely to develop diabetes, probably because fiber helps to delay stomach emptying, slowing the absorption of glucose into the bloodstream.

Indeed, a landmark review of nearly 20 years of research about carbohydrates and the role they play in health and disease concluded that at least 50 to 55 percent of daily calories should come from carbs. That's exactly the percentage of carbs you will be consuming in the *Eat Carbs, Lose Weight* food plan.

Pure Joy

Eating is about more than consuming the nutrients your body needs to function optimally. It's also about joy. Carbs add taste and texture to foods. I love biting into a slice of fresh whole-grain bread. I love the texture. It *feels* good to eat a bowl of whole-wheat pasta or a baked potato with a small pat of butter. When you give up the very foods you love the most, you miss out on the joy of eating.

The good news is that you can and should include all of your favorite foods on your weight-loss menu. As long as you follow a balanced diet, all foods—even chocolate—can help you lose weight. Even if you tend to crave and consequently overeat certain carbohydrate foods, you can feel confident about putting them back on your dinner plate or eating them for a snack. Chapter 3 will show you how.

CARBOHYDRATE ADDICTION

How to eat any high-carbohydrate food—including chocolate—without going overboard

I hear from many women who have tried low-carb diets—and hated them. These women tell me that cutting carbs from their diets makes them crave carbs more than ever. No matter whether they are trying Atkins or SugarBusters or something else, they find themselves smelling, staring at, and lusting for most of the high-carbohydrate foods they must walk past at the grocery store. Some women even tell me that they find themselves *dreaming* about carbs. They liken cutting back on carbs to trying to give up smoking.

Even more women—whether they have tried low-carb diets or not—tell me that they sometimes feel out of control when they see or smell certain types of carbohydrate foods. For example, some say that they don't think it will ever be possible to stop at just one cookie or a few tastes of cake. These women indulge in their guilty pleasures often and to an extreme. They don't stop at one slice of key lime pie. They eat the entire thing.

Such women often ask me whether I think it's possible to be *addicted* to carbs. The answer to that question is a complicated one. Many food researchers say that you can't form an addiction with a food like you can with a drug. A true addiction is an uncontrollable compulsion to repeat a behavior. When you are addicted, you not only crave more of something but also notice withdrawal symptoms when you don't indulge in your craving.

So, can eating a certain type of food cause an uncontrollable compulsion to eat more of it? Can ignoring a craving for a particular food result in withdrawal symptoms? It's possible. In the documentary *Super Size Me,* filmmaker Morgan Spurlock ate nothing but fast food for a month. As the consistent doses of fast food fattened his liver and spiked his blood cholesterol, a strange thing happened. Spurlock began noticing symptoms typical of addiction. Between meals, he felt fatigued and sick. Once he indulged in his fast-food fix, however, he felt energized. His doctors decided that, over the course of the month, he had become addicted to the high amounts of simple sugars and fat in fast food.

If it's possible to become addicted to fast food, then it seems equally plausible that one could become addicted to sugary, processed carbohydrate foods, especially chocolate. Some research seems to bear this out. In a study of 31 people completed at the University of Tampere in Finland, researchers tested the heart rates, salivation, and emotional responses of so-called chocolate addicts as well as nonaddicts. When the researchers placed chocolate in front of the participants, the "addicts" responded with increased heart rates and tended to overconsume the chocolate set before them, whereas the nonaddicts responded calmly and ate only a nibble or two.

Why do some people find sugary processed carbs so tempting, whereas others can see, smell, and even taste cake, chocolate, and other carbs and easily walk away from the dinner table? There are many good reasons why, as you will soon learn. The good news is this: No matter how out of control you feel around *any* food, you can take effective steps to reduce your cravings and get back in control of your eating. The *Eat Carbs, Lose Weight* plan will show you how.

"I Ate Carbs and Lost Weight!"

Name: Janice Orth

Age: 35

Town: Denver, Colorado

Weight Lost: 6 pounds in 4 weeks

Other Accomplishments: Feels a tremendous difference in her energy level, and her clothes fit more comfortably

"I have been overweight most of my life. During my grade-school years, I was not very active. I lost weight when I went to high school, but it was done the wrong way—by not eating. The pounds came back once I got married and started having children. After my second child, it took me 5 years to get down to my goal weight of 150 pounds, which I did by exercising.

"Then I became pregnant again. My little boy just turned one, and I'm still trying to lose the weight. My main motivation for starting *Eat Carbs, Lose Weight* was to have more energy. I want to stay healthy so that I can enjoy my children and my grandchildren in the future.

"I am thrilled with my results. I got the jump start I needed to start exercising again so I can eventually get down to my goal weight. I can definitely tell the difference in my energy level, and my clothes are fitting more comfortably. And other people have noticed a difference, too, telling me that I *look* more energized.

"I love the *Eat Carbs, Lose Weight* diet. The meals are very realistic and simple—and best of all, they taste wonderful. I will stick to using the meal plans while continuing down the road to better health.

"Having support from my family and from Denise really encouraged me and gave me the motivation to stick with the diet. My energy seems to grow daily, and I really want to thank Denise for helping me get started!"

Janice's advice: "Keep up your spirits and look at long-term goals. I have heard Denise say that the weight didn't just come on overnight, so we should not expect it to leave that way either. It takes commitment, but this diet is very simple and easy to follow . . . and it works!"

FOOD AS PLEASURE

Although many factors affect the strength of your cravings, the strongest among them centers on the levels of the neurotransmitter serotonin in your brain. Your brain houses a number of neurotransmitters, chemical messengers that relay important information from one neuron (or brain cell) to another. Among other things, levels of these messengers influence your mood, appetite, thoughts, and food cravings.

One of the neurotransmitters we discussed in chapter 2, serotonin, promotes feelings of joy, optimism, and calm. When serotonin levels are optimal, you sleep better, feel calmer, experience fewer cravings, and are less likely to overeat. On the other hand, when levels of this neurotransmitter drop too low, you may feel depressed and irritable, may crave sugary foods, and are more likely to overeat.

This may be why you find carbohydrates so addictive. When you feel sad or stressed, you may turn to carbs as if they were a drug. Once you eat some cookies or bread, you are rewarded with a rise in serotonin levels and feel calmer and happier as a result.

Sugary foods may reward you in yet another way: by lowering levels of the stress hormone cortisol. In one study, rats forced to swim in cold water (a stressful event for them) had lower cortisol levels when they drank sugar water compared with plain water.

You may also crave certain carbohydrate foods based on nostalgic memories of eating these foods in the past. When you go to a birthday party or wedding, for example, you may crave cake because you have eaten cake at these celebrations in the past and it reminds you of happy times. Similarly, you may crave mashed potatoes when you feel

Women and Cravings

Although the jury is still out regarding why, women are more likely than men to experience intense food cravings. About 97 percent of women, compared with 68 percent of men, report food cravings. Women give in to these cravings about half of the time, according to research conducted at the University of Calgary in Canada.

sad or depressed because they remind you of times during childhood when you felt safe and comforted.

Researchers suspect that chocolate may rank as the most highly craved carbohydrate food for a number of reasons. First and foremost, it tastes fantastic. Even a noncraver can admit that. Plus, chocolate's high sugar and fat content makes most people feel guilty when they eat it. As you'll soon learn, guilt will magnify a craving. Chocolate also contains many chemicals—including anandamines, caffeine, phenylethylamine, and magnesium—that act like drugs in the body. These chemicals can alter brain chemistry and disrupt behavior patterns. As with other types of carbohydrate, chocolate increases mood-boosting brain chemicals such as serotonin and dopamine. Chocolate also causes the brain to release more endorphins, the brain's natural painkillers.

OF CRAVERS AND NONCRAVERS

It may be hard to fathom, but not everyone has an equal affinity for carbohydrates. Just as drugs such as alcohol and nicotine affect different people in different ways, so do carbohydrates. As it turns out, some people tend to crave carbs, and some do not. In fact, researchers who conduct studies on cravings often split participants into two groups: carbohydrates cravers and non–carbohydrates cravers.

Researchers at the University of South Alabama noted that certain people "abuse carbs," eating them for their brain-altering properties instead of true hunger. In one of their studies, these researchers asked 113 male and 138 female college students to complete a questionnaire about the foods they craved and the moods they noticed after eating these foods. Students who labeled themselves as "carbohydrate cravers" said they felt distressed before their cravings and satisfied, happy, and relaxed after eating carbs, whereas the noncravers noticed no mood changes. The link between carbs and mood was strongest for those who craved sweets.

Research at the Massachusetts Institute of Technology also shows that different people respond differently to carbs. When noncravers eat sugary carbohydrates, they feel sleepy and depressed afterward. On the other hand, when carbohydrates cravers eat the same foods, they feel better.

Why do you lose control when you're around chocolate or sweets and your friend or office mate does not? Your brain may actually be wired differently, causing serotonin to not work as effectively. When serotonin levels are optimal, you have fewer cravings and are less likely to overeat. Researchers at MIT have found that carbohydrates cravers are more likely to feel angry and depressed than noncravers, an indication that low serotonin levels may be to blame.

Serotonin is also involved in sleep onset and pain sensitivity. In fact, some of the medications used to treat chronic pain syndromes, stress urinary incontinence, and insomnia optimize serotonin levels. Because of defective serotonin levels, the following types of people tend to crave carbohydrates.

Women with Premenstrual Syndrome (PMS)

Although many women complain of PMS every month, not all of them technically have this disorder. Originally described in 1931 by an American neurologist, true PMS includes the following four symptoms.

- Anxiety (irritability, sudden crying spells, anger, a sensation of being out of control)
- Depression (mental confusion, clumsiness, forgetfulness, paranoia, worry, suicidal thoughts)
- Cravings (usually for sweets or chocolate and sometimes for dairy products or alcohol)
- Heaviness (headache and fluid retention that causes weight gain, breast tenderness, and bloating)

About 70 percent of women do experience these symptoms, but only 30 to 40 percent experience symptoms severe enough to disrupt their normal routine. When symptoms become disabling, women are considered to have premenstrual dysphoric disorder (PMDD).

According to research at MIT, women with severe premenstrual syndrome increase their carbohydrate consumption by 24 percent during meals and 43 percent during snacks during the luteal phase of their cycle, roughly 2 weeks before menstruation. When they eat carbohydrates during this phase of the cycle, these women feel less tense and confused, happier, more energetic, and calmer. When they eat carbs during other phases of the cycle, however, women with severe PMS do not report these positive mental effects. Also, women who do not have severe PMS do not notice a mood boost from carbs during any phase of the cycle.

Although PMS is triggered by hormonal changes, the cravings for carbohydrates are probably brought on by low serotonin levels coupled with low blood sugar. The female hormone estrogen rises after menstruation and peaks at midcycle, during the luteal phase. As the estrogen builds, it increases fluid retention by as much as 5 pounds and causes a drop in blood sugar, which may bring on the cravings for sweets. It also drives down serotonin and endorphin levels. When researchers gave women a drug to boost levels of serotonin during this phase of the cycle, their cravings for carbs decreased.

There are some months when I experience a few symptoms of PMS, especially cravings, and I usually see a 2- to 3-pound fluctuation in my normal weight.

Men and Women with Depression

As with PMS, people who are depressed tend to have low levels of serotonin. Women are twice as likely to become depressed as men. Drugs that increase levels of serotonin tend to reduce carbohydrate binges in people with depression.

If you think you might be depressed, see your doctor for a diagnosis and medical advice. Your doctor may recommend a prescription medication that will help improve serotonin levels.

The Nonfood Cure for Cravings

Exercise may help alleviate symptoms of PMS by reducing stress and tension and elevating mood. It also improves blood circulation and increases the production of endorphins, natural feel-good brain chemicals.

In addition to following your doctor's advice and adopting a carb-smart strategy (see chapter 4), you can take a few additional nutritional steps to lift depression and reduce the cravings associated with it. First, take a daily multivitamin, as this simple tactic has been shown to help improve mood. (For advice on choosing your multi, see chapter 6.) Diets low in vitamin B_6 as well as a type of fat called omega-3 fatty acids may bring on or worsen depression. Below you'll find excellent food sources for these important nutrients.

Vitamin B_6: avocado, bananas, chicken, fish, green leafy vegetables, legumes, nuts

Omega-3s: fatty, cold-water fish such as salmon; fish-oil supplements; walnuts and walnut oil; flaxseeds, flaxseed meal, and flaxseed oil

Men and Women with Seasonal Affective Disorder (SAD)

Four times more common in women than men, this form of depression strikes in the winter, when the numbers of sunlight hours are at their lowest. Although the lack of sunlight and the accompanying blustery weather cause many people to crave comfort foods such as mashed potatoes, people with SAD tend to have more intense cravings than people without the disorder.

The term *seasonal affective disorder* was not coined until the early 1980s, but doctors have documented its symptoms as far back as the late 1800s. Common symptoms include the following: overeating and excessive weight gain, excessive sleeping, and cravings for sugary or starchy foods. People with SAD frequently experience a drop in immunity, an increase in tension or anxiety, and low sex drive as well. January and February usually mark the most difficult months for people with SAD.

Lack of sunlight during the winter months may affect the body's biological internal clock, lowering levels of serotonin. According to research, people with SAD may have lower levels of serotonin year-round. Then, when it drops even lower in the winter, these people experience acute and sometimes intense cravings for carbs. People with SAD may also have lower levels of the feel-good brain chemical dopamine that causes feelings of joy.

Eating carbs helps to raise levels of serotonin, which is why people with SAD crave these foods in the winter months. When researchers at MIT administered drugs to boost serotonin levels in people with SAD, cravings for carbs decreased.

If you think you might have SAD, see your doctor for a diagnosis and medical advice. The meal plan in *Eat Carbs, Lose Weight* will help stabilize serotonin levels. You'll be eating the right carbs, in the right amounts, at the right times to prevent cravings, binge-ing, and overeating. Also, the protein included in your meals will help to stabilize levels of dopamine.

Smokers Who Are Trying to Quit

Smokers tend to have lower serotonin levels than nonsmokers do. In fact, several researchers believe it's lower levels of this important brain chemical that addict some people to tobacco products, whereas others can try smoking and not get addicted.

Because nicotine raises levels of serotonin, quitting will lower levels of this brain chemical. This is one reason why smokers tend to become depressed and moody when they try to give up the habit. It's also one reason why they tend to gain weight. To make up for the loss in serotonin, many smokers overeat carbs.

If you smoke or use other types of tobacco products, talk to your family doctor about ways to help you quit. Your doctor might also recommend a nicotine replacement product such as the patch, counseling, a support group, or other options.

Say Goodbye to SAD

In addition to following the *Eat Carbs, Lose Weight* meal plan, you can take some other steps to reduce your cravings and boost your mood during the winter months. Try to get outside during the day to soak up some sunlight. For example, if you walk for fitness, take your walk during your lunch break. Also consider purchasing a light box designed for people with seasonal affective disorder. These white fluorescent lights mimic sunlight, tricking your brain into thinking that it isn't winter.

People with Diabetes or Prediabetes

Some research shows diabetes can increase your risk of depression. Although more research is needed to say for sure, it's possible people with diabetes have low levels of serotonin.

But diabetes may make you crave carbs for yet another reason. Because blood sugar remains chronically high, the body tends to overproduce the hormone insulin to try to bring blood sugar down. Among other things, high levels of insulin can make you hungry, particularly for carbs. With the right eating, exercise, and medical plan, however, you can get your diabetes under control. Once you do so, your cravings for carbs will decrease.

THE CRAVER'S DIET

In addition to your personal body chemistry, the way you eat can also affect your cravings. Veteran dieters, for example, tend to crave sweets, mostly because they are used to subsisting in a chronic low blood sugar state. Skipping meals or eating too few calories or carbohydrates will keep blood sugar low, causing your energy to plummet as your body quickly uses up the stored carbohydrate in your muscles. As blood sugar drops, your body will try to raise it by sending out a series of hormones that make you hungry for the foods most likely to raise blood sugar the fastest: quickly digestible starchy or sugary carbs. Indeed, when researchers in Edinburgh, Scotland, induced a low blood sugar state in 13 people with type 1 diabetes, the study participants were 65 percent more likely to experience intense food cravings—especially for high-carbohydrate foods—than when blood sugar levels were normal.

In addition to chronic dieting, stress and the lifestyle associated with it can cause you to eat in a way that increases your cravings for carbs. When you are feeling harried and hurried, you're more likely to grab easy-to-eat and easy-to-cook (or not cook at all) foods. Too often, these foods are full of sugar or processed starch. They spike blood

Are You a Carbohydrate Addict?

Take the following quiz to find out whether you are addicted to carbs.

1. Do you gain weight (more than 10 pounds) when you are under stress?
2. Have you ever been diagnosed with depression?
3. Have you ever been diagnosed with seasonal affective disorder (SAD)?
4. Do you tend to gain more than 10 pounds during the winter months?
5. Do you feel depressed and fatigued during the winter months?
6. Do you notice cravings for sweets during the winter but not during the spring and summer?
7. Have you ever been diagnosed with PMS or PMDD (premenstrual dysphoric disorder)?
8. Have you noticed the typical symptoms of PMS (heaviness, anxiety, depression, cravings) during the middle phase of your cycle?
9. If you are trying to quit smoking, do you tend to substitute carbohydrate foods in place of cigarettes?
10. Have you been diagnosed with diabetes or prediabetes?
11. When you crave carbohydrates, do your cravings usually surface in the afternoon or evening?
12. Do you tend to snack on mostly refined-carbohydrate foods such as dry breakfast cereal, bread or bagels, crackers, and cookies?
13. When you eat carbs, do you feel better shortly afterward?
14. Do you consume a third or more of your daily calories from carbs during unplanned snacking episodes?
15. Do you notice cravings for carbs more than once a week?
16. When you eat carbs, do you generally do so when you are not physically hungry?

If you answered yes to any of these questions, you may experience a tougher time resisting carbohydrates than someone who isn't a carbohydrates craver. The balanced meal plan in *Eat Carbs, Lose Weight* will help. So will the advice in this chapter and in chapter 4.

If you think you might have depression or seasonal affective disorder, see your medical doctor for help. If you continue to experience difficulty controlling your eating after following the advice in this chapter, consult with your physician and consider seeing a registered dietitian as well.

sugar levels, causing an overproduction of the hormone insulin. This drives down blood sugar too low, setting off more cravings.

HOW TO STOP THE CRAVINGS

If you follow the *Eat Carbs, Lose Weight* plan, your carbohydrate consumption will be 50 percent of your total daily calories. This ideal ratio will allow you to enjoy the carbohydrate foods you love *without* feeling any ill effects. You'll keep blood sugar levels stable, optimize the serotonin levels in your brain, feel satisfied after every meal and snack, and notice fewer cravings.

You'll also be eating the right carbs in the right balance at the right times. By spreading out your calorie intake through three meals and two snacks, you'll keep blood sugar levels stable, which will help lower cravings. You'll maximize your consumption of whole grains, fruits, vegetables, and legumes—carbohydrates that help stabilize blood sugar, turn down appetite, normalize serotonin levels, and prevent cravings. You'll minimize your consumption of refined foods and simple sugars—foods that turn up cravings. You'll also be getting a daily dose of exercise. In addition to blasting away stress and increasing levels of mood-boosting brain chemicals, daily exercise can help you to feel more confident, which improves your chances of sticking with your meal plan.

In her practice, nutritionist Amy Campbell has seen time and time again that cravings

The Midafternoon Doldrums

Carbohydrate cravings often hit during the middle of the afternoon, during the same time of day when the midafternoon slump tends to set in. This is when blood sugar levels drop, making you sluggish. (Another popular craving time is 9 P.M.) To prevent cravings from getting out of control in the mid to late afternoon, cut them off at the pass by *planning* on eating a midafternoon snack. The meal plan in *Eat Carbs, Lose Weight* includes two snacks every day: one in the morning and one in the afternoon. This will help to stabilize your blood sugar levels, reducing your cravings for sweets.

diminish greatly once her clients switch from a diet full of processed, high-glycemic, low-fiber foods to one that is low glycemic, minimally processed, and high in fiber. That said, you will still love your favorite foods. No diet will change your taste buds.

You can and should eat controlled servings of the foods you crave the most. If you crave a piece of chocolate but instead nibble on sliced fruit, you'll probably end up eating the sliced fruit *and* the chocolate. Trying to deny your craving will only strengthen

Making the Switch

Some carbs—such as the warm white bread served before your meal at a restaurant—are incredibly hard to resist. They are low in fiber, digest quickly, and send blood sugar soaring, especially when you eat them in the absence of other foods. You may find it difficult to hold yourself to just one serving—or two, or three.

Although they are not technically addictive, many of these carbohydrate foods can temporarily make you feel better psychologically by boosting levels of the feel-good brain chemical serotonin. This is one reason why we find them so tempting. True comfort foods, the following foods remind us of good times, celebrations, and warm family meals.

1. Chocolate

2. Ice cream

3. Cake

4. Cookies

5. White bread

6. Doughnuts

7. Pasta

8. Potato chips

If you can hold yourself to one serving of these foods, and really enjoy it, please do—and don't forget to congratulate yourself for listening to your cravings! But if you find you lose control when you eat these foods, try to satisfy your cravings with a healthier alternative. For example, instead of premium ice cream, would you feel just as satisfied with light ice cream, a frozen juice pop, or sorbet? Rather than fried potato chips, could you enjoy homemade baked ones just as much? Here are some better alternatives to turn to when cravings strike. Many of the following carbohydrate foods are high in fiber and low in fat and sugar. Your body will digest these foods slowly, stabilizing blood sugar levels.

1. Fresh fruit. This satisfies your sweet tooth while providing appetite-lowering fiber and health-promoting phytochemicals.

2. Vegetables. Eat them raw to satisfy your urge for something crunchy. If you must,

the craving. This is one reason why many people end their low-carb diets with a carbohydrate binge. After many weeks of denying themselves the foods they love the most, they eventually lose control and eat every carbohydrate food in sight.

So, once a day, indulge your taste buds with a small portion of one of your favorite foods. To eat the foods you love without going overboard, however, you must pay careful attention to the portions you put in your mouth. From chapter 1, you may remember that we humans tend to eat what we see. If you see an entire cake or pie, you'll want

sprinkle a little salt on top—try salt on sliced cucumber to simulate the experience of eating potato chips, for instance.

3. Yogurt. Although not high in fiber, yogurt is low in fat, packed with beneficial digestive bacteria, and satisfyingly sweet and creamy. It also provides some protein to turn down your appetite.

4. Nuts and seeds. Try these instead of potato chips when you feel an urge to crunch on something salty. The healthful fats and protein will lower your appetite before you can go overboard.

5. Popcorn. Go for the air-popped variety and sprinkle some Parmesan on top for a low-calorie, high-fiber crunch fest.

6. Whole-wheat pretzels. Better than their refined cousins, whole-wheat pretzels offer the crunch you desire, along with appetite-suppressing fiber.

7. Lower-fat string cheese. Although not high in fiber, this will hit your "cheese tooth" and is packed with protein for added staying power.

8. Rice or popcorn cakes. Studies show that these air-filled foods take up room in the stomach, making you feel fuller on fewer calories.

9. Soup. Opt for vegetable-packed, broth-based varieties. They are low in calories, high in fiber, and long on satisfaction.

10. Spicy foods (such as chili powder on popcorn). Spicy foods gently turn up the metabolism and turn down the appetite. You don't need to eat much to feel satisfied.

11. Baked sweet potato chips. Try this recipe: Mist sweet potato wedges with olive oil-flavored cooking spray and sprinkle with salt. Roast at 400°F for 40 minutes. Sprinkle with Parmesan cheese and bake 5 more minutes.

an entire cake or pie. On the other hand, if you see a small chocolate chip cookie, you'll savor that cookie and feel satisfied.

So, rather than stocking your cupboard with large bags of potato chips, for example, stock small individual servings instead. Instead of large chocolate bars, buy the miniatures that you usually hand out on Halloween.

You may notice that you eat many sugary, processed carbs somewhat mindlessly. Far from being your favorite foods, these sweet or crunchy carbs may merely have become a habit for you. You are used to eating them, therefore you crave them. Yet, if you really took the time to notice your reaction, you'd probably see that eating them doesn't satisfy you in the same way as eating your absolute favorite high-carbohydrate food—like premium ice cream or fresh-baked whole-grain bread—does.

For these junky processed foods, try to find a more suitable alternative that is high in fiber, low in glycemic load, and processed as little as possible. For example, can you switch from nutritionally bankrupt white bread to whole wheat? How about a satisfying baked sweet potato instead of potato chips that are packed with trans fats? (See "Making the Switch" on pages 60 and 61 for more ideas.) The more often you eat healthful carbs and minimize carbs that spike blood sugar, the easier it will be for you to indulge in your favorite high-quality foods from time to time, without losing control.

In addition to finding healthier carbohydrate options, use these tips to help reduce your cravings for refined carbohydrate foods.

Never vilify a food—no matter how decadent. When Shippensburg University researcher Debra Zellner, Ph.D., studied the chocolate cravings of American and Spanish women, she concluded that many American women crave chocolate simply because they see the food as a nutritional taboo. Spanish women, on the other hand, don't experience cravings for chocolate but rather for cola—a drink they consider a nutritional taboo. As it turns out, feeling guilty about eating a food—any food—can cause you to lose control. So rather than telling yourself that you are "being bad" by indulging in chocolate or any other guilty pleasure, congratulate yourself for honoring your craving.

Eat a daily serving of green leafy vegetables. In addition to boosting your consumption of appetite-lowering fiber, you'll also consume plenty of folate. A deficiency in this B vitamin has been linked with depression, which can heighten food cravings.

Eat at regular 3- to 4-hour intervals. The *Eat Carbs, Lose Weight* plan includes three meals and two snacks for a reason. Besides helping to keep you feeling satisfied during the day on fewer calories, this will also stabilize blood sugar levels. Because these meals and snacks are low in sugar, they will also help to lift the symptoms of PMS, particularly the headache and fatigue.

Cut back on sugar. In addition to reducing cravings, this will help to reduce the bloating, fatigue, tension, and depression associated with PMS. See chapter 4 for tips on reducing your sugar consumption.

Eat balanced meals. The menus in *Eat Carbs, Lose Weight* include balanced portions of carbohydrates, protein, and fat. The protein and fat help ease the entry of glucose into your bloodstream, stabilizing blood glucose and insulin levels. They also help you to feel satisfied after eating and less hungry later in the day.

Find an outlet for your mood. Instead of turning to food, go for a walk, talk to a friend, write in a journal, or get a massage. Find noncaloric ways to soothe yourself and boost your mood.

EATING CARB SMART

How eating the right carbs will rein in your cravings for the wrong ones

During the 1980s and 1990s, many of us—including me—believed that all carbohydrates were healthy and that all fats were, well, fattening.

We now know that this type of thinking is a giant oversimplification. As I mentioned in chapter 1, many people *gained* weight during the low-fat years. As it turns out, not all fats are bad and not all carbs are good. The monounsaturated fats found in avocado and olive oil, for example, and the omega-3 fatty acids found in fish and nuts may improve heart health, fend off cancer, and possibly even drive down appetite and enhance brain health. Some carbohydrates, such as those made from processed white flour and sugar, can do the opposite: increase the risk for heart disease, cause you to overeat, and possibly even set the stage for cancer.

We can thank the low-carbohydrate movement for this new, more informed view of fats and carbs. Many low-carb diets were the first to point out the negative effects of some types of carbohydrates. Although these diets take matters to an unnecessary extreme, they have helped to educate us all about the fundamentals of which carbohydrates to minimize in our diets.

In this chapter, you will find four carb-smart tactics designed to help you go a few steps further: You'll not only learn to minimize your consumption of weight-promoting carbs but also learn to maximize your consumption of weight-loss-friendly carbs. Following these carb-smart strategies will help you to reduce your cravings for unhealthful carbs, boost your energy, and feel more satisfied after every meal.

NOT AS SIMPLE AS WE ONCE THOUGHT

You have heard me talk about the difference between simple and complex carbohydrates. Simple carbs are simple sugars—including white table sugar (called sucrose), the sugar found in fruit (fructose), and the sugar found in milk (lactose). You'll also find simple carbs in many processed foods in the form of high-fructose corn syrup.

Complex carbs include starches and fiber. They are called complex because they include three or more glucose units per molecule. (Simple carbs contain just one or two.) Foods such as potatoes, bread, pasta, vegetables, and beans are all examples of complex carbohydrates.

For many years, we were taught to minimize simple carbs and maximize complex carbs. The theory went like this: Simple carbs—found predominantly in soft drinks and candy—offered us mostly empty calories. They also could pass directly from the intes-

Stop the Deprivation

Although you do want to cut back on unhealthful carbohydrates such as processed, low-fiber foods and foods with added sugars, you need not give up such foods entirely. If you love the occasional piece of cake or the occasional soft drink, that's fine. Just don't go overboard. Telling yourself that you are not allowed to consume such foods will make you crave them even more. Try to strike a balance between weight-loss-promoting carbs and weight-gain-promoting ones. For example, try to hold your consumption of high-glycemic, low-fiber, processed carbs to only 10 percent of your total daily calories. The meal plans found in this book do just that.

tine into the bloodstream without getting broken down by digestive enzymes. Complex carbs, on the other hand, had to first get broken down into single sugar molecules before getting absorbed into the bloodstream. Some scientists thought that simple carbs therefore provided quick but fleeting energy. These carbs drove blood sugar up too quickly, causing the body to overproduce insulin and consequently lower blood sugar too quickly, resulting in hunger and fatigue. Complex carbs, because they took longer to reach the bloodstream, provided better, lasting energy.

At least, that's the theory. Although this theory may hold true for some simple carbs and some complex carbs, it doesn't hold true for all of them. In the late 1970s, David Jenkins and other researchers at St. Michael's Hospital in Toronto began testing how various carbohydrates—both simple and complex—affected blood sugar levels. They compared the foods they tested with the speed at which white bread affected blood sugar, giving white bread a score of 100. If a food turned into blood sugar faster than white bread, they gave it a score higher than 100. If it hit the bloodstream more slowly, they gave it a score below 100.

They—and much of the scientific community—were surprised by their results, which the researchers published as the Glycemic Index in the *American Journal of Clinical Nutrition* in 1981. For example, instant rice, a complex carb, had a high glycemic index of 124—higher than table sugar, a simple carb. Cornflakes, couscous, and instant oatmeal, all complex carbs, also ranked higher than sugar. As it turned out, the effect of foods on blood sugar was much more complex than previously thought.

CARB-SMART TACTIC #1: CHOOSE SLOW CARBS OVER FAST CARBS

Since the early 1980s, researchers have conducted many studies on the glycemic index (GI). Not only have they tested hundreds of additional foods and assigned them glycemic ratings, they've also looked at the health effects of high- and low-glycemic diets.

Research consistently shows, for example, that people tend to feel less full and con-

"I Ate Carbs and Lost Weight!"

Name: Elizabeth Lane
Age: 34
Town: Houston, Texas
Weight Lost: 4 pounds in 4 weeks
Other Accomplishments: Got started in the right direction and set clearer health goals

"My husband loves me unconditionally, which is wonderful, but unfortunately this has also allowed me to steadily gain weight since I married him in 2001. I am not obese, but I have reached a size 12 and refuse to go any higher.

"I have tried many diets, most which I have found in women's magazines, but either they became too boring or the meals were unrealistic. I don't think it should cost a fortune to follow a diet.

"I was attracted to *Eat Carbs, Lose Weight* because Denise Austin has always been a role model for me. In my teens, I purchased a cassette tape and instruction booklet of hers called *Hot Legs,* and I have kept it all these years because the workout was so well balanced. Denise is an inspiring person.

"The diet was everything I expected from Denise. I found the foods were very tasty and easy to make. I usually have cravings, but on the plan I forgot about them. It's amazing how the mind creates false hungers.

"My energy level also went up, and I found it easier to take that 15-minute break from work to walk the tunnel system here in downtown Houston.

"Although I only lost 4 pounds and ½ inch from my waist, I gained muscle, so I think my fat loss was more significant than it looks on paper. My mother, who always helps me keep it real, noticed my weight loss right away.

"Overall, I feel really good about what I've achieved. This jump start has gotten me going in the right direction. God willing, I will take this lesson and continue to move forward with the health goals I've set for myself."

Elizabeth's advice: "First, eliminate fast food and soda. Set daily goals for yourself and keep them simple and easy to follow. Leave fruit lying on the counter so you can grab it on the run (a piece of fruit on the way out the door in the morning can become that breakfast you would have skipped). Don't deprive yourself, but be aware that what you put in your body affects everything."

sequently eat more after consuming high-GI foods compared with low-GI foods. One study completed at the University of Sydney in Australia found low-GI diets produce greater weight loss than high-GI diets, even when the number of daily calories is the same. When researchers fed animals diets rich in high-GI starches, the animals gained weight and produced more enzymes that promoted fat storage. In a separate study of pregnant women, a high-GI diet resulted in greater weight at term than a low-GI diet.

A diet composed primarily of high-GI foods may also be bad for your health. Studies done at Harvard have found that people who eat high-GI foods most of the time are more at risk for heart disease and diabetes than people who consume mostly low-GI foods. Harvard's Nurses' Health Study, for example, examined the diets of more than 80,000 nurses. This study found that replacing polyunsaturated fat with high-glycemic carbs increased the risk of heart disease by more than 50 percent. Other research has shown that diets high in quickly digested added sugars worsen blood cholesterol, boost triglyceride levels, and decrease blood sugar control. Food scientists around the world consider the glycemic index so important for both health and weight loss that the World Health Organization has recommended that labels list a food's GI value.

As I mentioned in chapter 1, however, the glycemic index doesn't always tell the whole story. Some foods—such as carrots, watermelon, and pumpkin—rate high on the index but don't necessarily dramatically raise blood sugar levels. Although your body digests these foods quickly, they don't contain enough carbohydrate calories to greatly affect blood sugar.

Need a Mood Boost? Eat Carb Smart

In chapter 2, I told you that you must consume carbohydrates to maintain an optimal mood. Low-glycemic-index carbohydrates that come from high-fiber, whole-grain foods provide your best sources of mood-boosting carbs. Because the carbohydrates from these foods enter the bloodstream slowly, they hold insulin levels steady. This allows the amino acid tryptophan smooth access into your brain for a longer period of time, providing a long-lasting boost of the feel-good neurotransmitter serotonin.

A more useful measure of fast and slow carbs is the glycemic load (GL), which we defined in chapter 1. It may help to understand the difference between GI and GL by thinking about wine. Each sip from the glass of wine contains the same percentage of alcohol. How much alcohol actually enters your bloodstream, on the other hand, depends on how much wine you drink. Have just a few sips and you notice no ill consequences. Drink the whole glass and refill it a couple of times and you'll probably get a bit tipsy. Like those first sips of wine, a high-GI food does not necessarily raise blood sugar very high if you don't eat that much of it, and therefore it will provide only a small glycemic load of carbohydrate for your body to process.

Although slow carbs are definitely better for weight loss, you need not research the glycemic index or glycemic load of every food you eat. First of all, we've already done this math for you. The meals in *Eat Carbs, Lose Weight* are all low in glycemic load. Second, once you have a basic understanding of the factors that influence a food's glycemic index and load, you can easily tell whether a food contains fast or slow carbohydrates, without having to look up the specific index or load of those foods. Finally, researchers haven't tested the glycemic values for every single food, so understanding what affects a food's glycemic nature will help you to consistently eat smarter than looking up the glycemic value of every food you eat. (Still, if you're curious for a few examples, check out "How the Glycemic Index Compares with the Glycemic Load," on pages 70 and 71.)

A number of factors affect the glycemic index of a food. They include the type of sugar used to form the carbohydrate, the type of starch (some starches are more readily digestible than others), the way the food was cooked or processed, and other nutrients in the food such as fat or protein. To choose low-GI foods most of the time, follow these pointers.

Opt for slow-cooking foods. To make many instant foods, food manufacturers chop up grains such as rice and oats into very fine particles. This not only speeds up the cooking time but also speeds the transit of sugar into your bloodstream. Although it may take 45 minutes to cook brown rice—which has a much lower index than instant white rice—it's worth the extra time when it comes to losing weight and keeping it off.

Choose processed carbohydrate foods that contain at least 3 to 5 grams of fiber per serving. Fiber helps to slow digestion, easing the entrance of sugar into the bloodstream. When sugar enters the bloodstream more slowly, blood sugar levels remain more con-

How the Glycemic Index Compares with the Glycemic Load

As you can see by examining the following chart, a high glycemic index (GI) does not necessarily translate into a high glycemic load (GL).

✧ A low GI rating = 55 or less; a medium GI rating = 56 to 69; a high GI rating = 70 to 100.

✧ A low GL rating = 10 or less; a medium GL rating = 11 to 19; a high GL rating = 20 or more.

If you are curious about the glycemic load or glycemic index of different foods, go to the University of Sydney's Web site, www.glycemicindex.com. Here you can plug hundreds of foods into the site's calculator, and it will compute the load and index values for you.

Food	Glycemic Index	Glycemic Load
Peanuts	23	1
Sausage	28	1.5
Peas	22	2.5
Oat bran (raw)	59	3
Microwave popcorn	55	3.5
Chocolate milk (low-fat)	24	4
Watermelon	72	4.3
Pears, canned	43	4.5
Apple	34	5
Lentils	52	5.5
Sourdough rye	48	6.5
Chocolate ice cream	68	6.7
All-Bran cereal	38	7

sistent. Fiber offers many other important weight-loss benefits, which is why I've named it Carb-Smart Tactic #2.

Eat high-glycemic foods with a little fat or protein. Both fat and protein slow digestion. If you want to eat a highly processed, low-fiber food, consuming it with a little fat

Food	Glycemic Index	Glycemic Load
Dried apricots	32	8
Oatmeal cookies	54	8.5
All Sport (orange)	53	9
Maple syrup	54	9.5
Banana	42	10
Sweet corn	62	10
Salmon sushi	48	10.5
Corn chips	42	11
White chocolate	44	12
Bran muffin	60	12.5
Sweet potato	48	12.5
Milk chocolate	42	13
Doughnut	76	14.3
Meat ravioli	39	15
White rice	38	16
Pretzels	83	16.1
Baked potato	78	17
Shredded wheat	83	18
Froot Loops	69	18
Linguine	43	19
Corn Pops cereal	80	21.5
Chocolate cake	38	22

or protein will help to slow the transport of sugar into the bloodstream. For example, if you love instant white rice, eat it as part of a stir-fry that includes chicken, shrimp, or other lean protein foods. If you love white bread, try dipping it in olive oil first.

CARB-SMART TACTIC #2: CHOOSE HIGH-FIBER FOODS OVER LOW-FIBER FOODS

In chapter 2, you learned about many of the benefits of fiber. Fiber helps to slow digestion, stabilizes blood sugar, and allows you to feel satisfied on fewer calories. One large-scale study found that women who consumed the most fiber in their diets were 49 percent less likely to gain weight over a period of 12 years than women who consumed the least amount of fiber.

Most people consume 10 to 15 grams of fiber a day, but you need much more than that—at least 20 grams, but better to get up to 35 grams—to improve digestion, feel satisfied on fewer calories, and remain healthy. Here are some easy ways to increase your fiber consumption.

Don't peel fruits and vegetables. Because fiber forms the outer cell walls of plants, it tends to be housed in the outer covering of carbohydrate foods. For example, half of the fiber in a baked potato is in the skin. Similarly, a third of the fiber of an apple is in the skin.

How to Tell If a Food Is Really Whole Grain

Many food products try to masquerade as healthy. For example, "wheat bread" often has a brown tint to it that comes from food coloring. It's really white bread. After all, technically, white flour still comes from wheat. Also, "multigrain" bread may indeed include many grains, but they all may be refined. Finally, many pasta products boast that they contain semolina or durum wheat flour. These flours are still refined. A true whole-grain product uses a whole grain such as whole wheat, whole rye, or whole oats as a main ingredient (the first or one of the first few listed on the ingredient list).

Choose a breakfast cereal that contains at least 3 to 5 grams of fiber and top it with fresh fruit. Your fruit will add another 1 or 2 grams of fiber to your cereal. Cold cereals vary wildly in fiber content, from almost zero to 12 or 13 grams per serving. The highest in fiber aren't always the most palatable, however, which is why Harvard nutritionist Amy Campbell and I recommend 3 to 5 grams. Many of the most delicious brands land right about there.

Keep frozen vegetables such as peas and spinach well stocked in your freezer. No matter what recipe you are making, whether it's a stir-fry or a pot of soup, ask yourself whether you can add more vegetables. Chances are you can, and the more veggies you add, the more fiber your meal will contain. In addition to frozen vegetables, try adding grated carrots, zucchini, or cabbage to chili, meatloaf, and other casseroles in place of some of the meat.

Keep canned beans in your cupboard. This allows you to quickly and easily add beans to salads, soups, rice, and many other dishes. Don't forget—beans are a great source of oligosaccharides, the complex sugars that help stabilize blood sugar and reduce your appetite.

Snack on raw vegetables. If you are looking for some crunch, try chopped carrots or sliced cucumbers, radishes, or turnips. You can even sprinkle them with a tiny bit of salt to simulate the taste of your favorite crunchy snack food.

Steam or stir-fry vegetables instead of boiling them. When you boil a vegetable too long, you may lose some of the fiber in the water. And besides—who wants to eat mushy veggies?

CARB-SMART TACTIC #3: CHOOSE WHOLE FOODS OVER REFINED

Grains come from seeds of plants that are in the grass family. For example, wheat—possibly the most well-known grain—comes from seeds on top of wheatgrass. Other grains include rye, barley, rice, corn, and oats. When intact, a grain seed contains three parts:

an outer layer of bran, a middle layer called an endosperm, and a nutrient-rich inner layer called the germ. Whole-grain foods contain all of these layers, whereas refined foods tend to house only the endosperm, the part of the seed that is richest in starch and lowest in fiber.

This refining process makes the grain easier to digest. So, after you eat a refined grain—such as instant white rice—your blood sugar levels will rise more dramatically than after eating a whole grain, such as brown rice. The fiber housed in whole-grain foods may influence gut hormones that make you feel full after eating. Research has

Make the Whole-Grain Switch

Just about all of your favorite carbohydrate foods are sold in two ways: refined and whole. The more often you choose the whole variety, the better your chances of weight-loss success. Make the following switches.

Instead of . . .	Try . . .
White bread	100 percent whole-wheat bread such as the Baker's Inn brand. In addition to being 100 percent whole grain, Baker's Inn contains no high-fructose corn syrup. It also offers 5 grams of protein per slice.
Refined pasta	A blend made from 50 percent whole wheat and 50 percent white flour, such as Ronzoni Healthy Harvest. This half-and-half blend is a step up from refined pasta but not as chewy in texture as 100 percent whole-wheat pasta.
White rice	Slow-cooking brown rice.
Instant oatmeal	Steel-cut oats, such as McCann's Irish Oatmeal.
Pearled barley	Hulled barley, which contains the germ and bran of the barley seed. Pearled barley contains only the endosperm.

consistently shown that people who eat more whole-grain foods weigh less than people who consume more refined grains. In one study completed at the University of Sydney, researchers tested seven different types of bread for how well the bread filled people up and prevented them from snacking later in the day. White bread resulted in the least satiety among all of the types of bread.

In addition to fiber, whole grains also offer additional phytonutrients, vitamins, and minerals that are good for your health. For example, unlike refined grains, whole grains are a rich source of vitamin E, selenium, magnesium, folate, and potassium, all of which may help fend off heart disease. The respected Insulin Resistance Arteriosclerosis Study suggests that cutting back on refined grains and replacing them with whole can improve insulin sensitivity. Insulin resistance has been linked to high blood pressure, heart disease, high levels of blood fats called triglycerides, low levels of healthy HDL cholesterol, and some cancers. It's often a precursor to type 2 diabetes.

To consume more whole grains, do the following:

✧ When purchasing packaged foods such as breakfast cereal, commercially baked bread, and crackers, check the ingredients list to see if a "whole" grain such as whole oats or whole wheat is listed first on the label.

✧ Look for the following claim on food packaging: "Diets rich in whole-grain foods and other plant foods and low in total fat, saturated fat, and cholesterol may reduce the risk for heart disease and certain cancers." For manufacturers to make that claim on their packaging, the Food and Drug Administration requires whole-grain products to include at least 51 percent whole grain by weight.

✧ Choose cereals, breads, and other grain products that offer 3 to 5 grams of fiber per serving. Because the fiber in a grain is housed in the outer shell, foods that contain more fiber tend to be less refined than foods that contain less fiber. Some of the tastiest brands include a mix of numerous whole grains.

✧ Add whole grains such as barley, brown rice, and whole-wheat pasta to soups, stews, and other dishes.

◇ Eat air-popped popcorn as a snack. (Yep, it's a whole grain!)

◇ Experiment with new grains that you may not have tried before, such as bulgur or quinoa. (See "The Whole Picture" for a list of alternative grains.)

◇ When you bake bread and other foods, substitute whole-wheat flour for up to half of the white flour in a recipe.

◇ Top casseroles with wheat germ or whole-wheat bread crumbs.

CARB-SMART TACTIC #4: CUT BACK ON ADDED SUGARS

You may only think of added sugars as the white stuff you scoop out of your sugar bowl. Yet, table sugar probably accounts for only a small percentage of the sugar you consume in a typical day.

Some of the most obvious places—such as soft drinks and cookies—are only the tip of the added-sugar iceberg. You'll find sugar lurking in many unexpected places, ranging from pasta sauce and salad dressing to energy bars and ketchup. The World Health Organization recommends we consume no more than 10 percent of our daily calories

The Whole Picture

Wheat is probably the most well-known grain, but you have many more grains from which to choose. They include:

Amaranth	Millet
Barley	Oats
Brown rice	Quinoa
Buckwheat (kasha)	Rye
Corn	Spelt
Bulgur	Wild rice
Flaxseed	

from added sugars, which translates to about 100 to 200 calories. That's the amount in just one 16-ounce bottle of Coke.

Most Americans consume much more than 10 percent. The U.S. Department of Agriculture estimates that the typical American consumes 147 pounds of sugar per year, up from 113 pounds per person in 1966. That's more like 16 percent per day.

All of this adds up to plenty of excess calories from sugar. Worse, the type of sugar used to sweeten many processed foods—high-fructose corn syrup—may be worse for your health and your waistline than table sugar. In 1966, no foods contained this sweetener, but in 2001, the typical person consumed 62 pounds of it a year. Indeed, consumption of high-fructose corn syrup increased 1,000 percent between 1970 and 1990—consumption of no other food or food group has increased that quickly! That comes to about 132 calories of corn syrup a day for the average adult. Some people consume as much as 316 calories of this sweetener a day, according to research completed at Louisiana State University's Pennington Biomedical Research Center in Baton Rouge.

Made from cornstarch, corn syrup is a thick liquid that tastes sweeter than refined sugar, making it less costly for food manufacturers to sweeten their foods. It's also easier to blend into beverages, which is why it has become the sweetener of choice in soft drinks and fruit-flavored beverages.

Researchers at Louisiana State believe that the human body treats high-fructose corn syrup differently than it does table sugar. When you consume table sugar, a number of biochemical reactions take place in your body that signal you to stop eating. For example, levels of the hormone leptin rise, and levels of another hormone, ghrelin, drop. This turns down your appetite.

But unlike table sugar, high-fructose corn syrup does not trigger this hormonal reaction. In theory, the absence of this biochemical reaction could cause you to overeat, because your brain doesn't recognize that calories have just come in. Although this theory has yet to be tested in the lab, the increase in corn syrup consumption from 1966 to the current day exactly mirrors a dramatic increase in obesity.

In addition to probably promoting weight gain, this sugar may also be bad for your health. The liver converts high-fructose corn syrup into a type of blood fat called triglycerides more easily than it does glucose. High levels of this blood fat have been linked to heart disease. In studies done on rats, researchers at the University of California, Davis, have linked high consumption of this sweetener to insulin resistance, high triglyceride

What about Sugar Substitutes?

Let me tell you right up front, I don't like to use artificial sweeteners. I think they have an aftertaste. In general, with all my food, I like to go as close to the source as possible—and I like to keep it natural. I prefer butter to margarine, fresh to processed, organic to those foods grown with pesticides. And sweets are no exception.

The only artificial sweeteners you'll find on the *Eat Carbs, Lose Weight* menu plan are in the light yogurt. All the recipes, meals, snacks, and desserts are prepared using sugar, honey, or fruit juice as sweeteners.

That said, when used sparingly, sugar substitutes such as NutraSweet and Splenda allow you to indulge in sweet tastes without the calories or sky-high blood sugar. Yet, not all of these artificial sweeteners affect your metabolism and health the same way. Most sweeteners, such as Equal, Splenda, and Sweet'n Low, contain no calories and do not affect blood sugar levels. However, a type of artificial sweetener commonly found in products marketed as "low carb" and in sugar-free candy does contain calories (about 2 calories per gram versus table sugar's 4 calories per gram) and, thus, will raise your blood sugar.

These sweeteners, called sugar alcohols, are found in the list of ingredients under the names sorbitol, mannitol, and xylitol. Although low-carb products claim these sugars don't count, they certainly do. In addition to raising blood sugar and contributing excess calories to your diet, they also may cause cramping, gas, and diarrhea—not exactly the experience you're looking for from a "chocolate" treat.

Although diet soda is definitely better than the real thing in terms of calories and blood sugar levels, you do have other options. When I'm thirsty, I always turn to water, green tea, or herbal tea first. These beverages all contain zero calories and have powerful health benefits, too. Even better, they don't result in undesirable side effects such as diarrhea. Next on my list is diluted fruit juice.

levels, and high blood pressure. A study published in the *American Journal of Clinical Nutrition* in 2004 linked the consumption of high-fructose corn syrup to type 2 diabetes, especially when fiber consumption was low. Further research done by the U.S. Department of Agriculture suggests that high-fructose corn syrup may play a role in bone loss. Until the final verdict is in, why not play it safe and just avoid it? You'll be much better off without.

Here are some ways to reduce your consumption of added sugars.

⬧ Choose canned fruit that's packed in water instead of heavy syrup.

Stay Fluid

I'm a big believer in drinking at least eight glasses of water a day. Staying hydrated helps you stay energetic. When you become dehydrated, your blood actually thickens. This makes your heart beat harder—and more often—to push blood through your vessels. End result: You feel tired. Drinking plenty of water also can help lower your appetite, as water can weigh down the stomach and help you to feel full.

When it comes to eating carb smart, however, water offers yet another bonus: It helps to keep fiber moving through your intestines. When you suddenly increase your fiber intake, an unwelcome consequence can be bloating and gas. Over time, your intestinal flora will get used to the increase in fiber, and the bloating and gas will subside. In the meantime, however, you can ease matters by drinking enough water. When you are well hydrated, fiber absorbs more water in the intestine, which helps soften stool, allowing it to move through your intestine more quickly.

Many of us can easily become dehydrated without even noticing. How about that day-long shopping spree? How much water did you drink? What about that road trip you took? How many glasses of water did you drink in the car?

To help ensure that I consume plenty of water, particularly when I'm away from home, I stock bottled waters in just about every conceivable location I might find myself. I have them in my car, in my purse, on my desk—everywhere. This way, I never find myself stranded without some water to drink. Plus, having them everywhere is an easy reminder to drink more water.

✧ Experiment with natural sweeteners such as cinnamon, cardamom, and vanilla. Try them instead of sugar on hot cereal, in yogurt, and in your tea.

✧ Switch from "fruit-flavored" beverages and "juice drinks"—which are packed with high-fructose corn syrup and no real fruit juice—to diluted 100 percent fruit juice such as pomegranate juice, guava juice, and papaya juice. Goya makes many different juices. I like to drink a different one with breakfast each day. For any time of day, I mix roughly half a shot glass of one of these juices with seltzer or club soda for a tasty, low-sugar, refreshing drink.

✧ Cut back on your consumption of soft drinks sweetened with high-fructose corn syrup. Instead, drink diet soft drinks (only if you have to—I don't), diluted fruit juice (better), or water (best).

✧ Read food labels to find out if a product contains added sugars. Look for the words *high-fructose corn syrup, corn syrup, molasses, honey, fruit juice concentrate, cane sugar, brown sugar,* and *raw sugar.* Choose foods that list sugar (by any of these names) fifth or later on the ingredient list. (And, in general, stay away from ingredient lists with words you can't pronounce or understand!)

✧ Switch from heavily sweetened breakfast cereals (which are really more like candy than food) to whole grain.

✧ Buy plain yogurt and mix in real fruit instead of eating fruit-flavored yogurts.

✧ Limit reduced-fat and fat-free products. To make these products palatable, food manufacturers generally replace the fat with added sugars.

THE *EAT CARBS, LOSE WEIGHT* FITNESS PLAN

You'll love this 12-minute total body blast

By now, I hope you are thrilled to welcome carbs back into your life. Once you start eating the right carbs in balanced portions, you will experience dramatic and exciting results. You will not only shed fat and reduce your cravings but also increase your energy levels, boost your mood, and feel better about yourself and your life.

Can you imagine life getting any better than that? Well, it can. Once you combine the *Eat Carbs* nutrition plan with the *Eat Carbs* fitness plan, you will see your results take on a new dimension. In just 12 simple moves, you'll tone up from head to toe, sculpting and slimming your thighs, buns, hips, tummy, arms, and back. And with a strong and toned body, you'll also experience renewed energy. You'll spring out of bed each morning ready to tackle the day. You'll glow with a vibrancy that only comes from regular exercise.

Best of all, you can accomplish all of this in just 12 minutes a day. The daily exercise routine in the *Eat Carbs* plan is short, but don't let that fool you. Although 12 minutes is the absolute minimum amount of time you can spend exercising, you will definitely see results if you spend those 12 minutes wisely. With the 12-minute Daily Dozen routine, you will. Each day, you will complete 12 moves that will strengthen muscles in your arms, chest, back, legs, tummy, and buttocks.

Many diets promise fast results with no exercise. Such claims are certainly enticing, but they simply aren't accurate. As I've mentioned before, you can lose weight on *any* diet by eating fewer calories. It doesn't matter whether the diet includes only grapefruit or cabbage soup or protein foods. If you eat fewer calories than you burn, you *will* lose weight.

Here's the catch. You will eventually hit a plateau and then gain back the weight. In fact, you'll probably gain more than you lost in the first place. Dietary changes are not enough to lose weight and keep it off. You must add exercise to your weight-loss formula for optimum success. It's about calories in, calories out.

Exercise helps you lose weight and keep it off by preserving your metabolism. When you restrict calories without exercising, your fat cells send signals to your brain, saying, "Famine! Enter survival mode." Your brain responds by ordering your fat-storing enzymes to increase. Eventually, you hit a plateau because these enzymes make it harder and harder for your body to release and get rid of fat.

In addition to increasing your fat-storing enzymes, dieting without exercise also tends to cause your body to cannibalize muscle protein for fuel. Rather than losing weight from where you want—your fat stores—you lose weight from where you don't—your muscle protein. Although you want to lose the fat, you don't want to lose the muscle. Every pound of muscle burns up to 50 calories a day as it busily processes proteins. When you lose muscle, your metabolism slows down and you burn fewer calories. So when you go off your diet, your body is burning fewer calories—as many as 250 fewer calories a day—and has a higher amount of fat-storing enzymes.

So you end up on a dieting roller coaster, a never-ending process of cutting calories, losing fat, slowing your metabolism, and gaining back even more fat. Each time you try to lose weight, your efforts will feel even more difficult.

You should add exercise to your weight-loss formula for another important reason: It's good for you. Completing strengthening exercises—such as the ones suggested in the routine in this chapter—helps not only to build muscle and bolster your metabolism but also to preserve bone mass. Daily exercise also can lower blood pressure and cholesterol, increase your energy, and help you to feel and look younger.

According to the National Weight Control Registry—a database full of facts about thousands of people who have lost 30 or more pounds and kept it off for more than a year—exercise provides a crucial ingredient to any successful weight-loss plan. Nearly all of the successful maintainers on the National Weight Control Registry exercised both to lose weight and to keep it off. For many, it wasn't until they added exercise to the mix that they were able to not only lose weight but keep it off for good.

YOUR MINIMUM DAILY DOSE

Exercise is so important to your success that I decided to create an excuse-proof plan. I wanted every single person who picked up this book to look at this exercise plan and think, "Now that's a plan I can do."

To sculpt lean muscle and burn fat, you will combine my 12-minute Daily Dozen routine with regular walking. Plus, you won't need to go out and buy any new exercise equipment, though I do suggest a good supportive walking shoe. This way, you can exercise anywhere at any time. As long as you have your body with you, you can fit in your workout for the day. It doesn't get any more convenient than this.

You'll soon learn more about the simple 12-minute routine that I designed to sculpt sexy muscle and rev up your metabolism. Before we get to that, let's talk about your walking program. I'd like you to walk 3 or 4 days a week for at least 30 minutes. This is the amount of exercise the National Institutes of Health recommends for optimum health.

Cardiovascular exercise, such as walking, both conditions your heart and tricks your body into burning more fat as fuel. Walking is my favorite form of cardiovascular exercise because it's easy on the joints and incredibly convenient. But I believe that any cardio workout is great: aerobics, stairclimbers, elliptical trainers, swimming.

If you have never walked for fitness before, start with a 10-minute walk and work up to 30 minutes from there. Personally, I like to walk in the morning. That way, I've gotten my exercise out of the way before the phone starts ringing and various time commitments start calling. If you're not a morning person, try taking a walk during your lunch break. Or take one as soon as you get home from work. Make it a regular routine.

In addition to your cardio walk, each day try to take more steps during your daily tasks than you did the day before. For example, make it a regular habit to take the stairs instead of the elevator and to walk into the bank rather than use the drive-thru. Consider wearing a pedometer, an inexpensive device that you attach to your waistband to record the number of steps you take in a day. Make 10,000 steps per day your goal.

SIMPLE, EASY, AND EFFECTIVE

The following 12 moves are your "minimum daily exercise requirement." This head-to-toe routine should be performed in the sequence shown. It's easy. You can do this!

The *Eat Carbs, Lose Weight* fitness routine includes a blend of my favorite yoga, Pilates, and strength movements. It's convenient, fast, gentle on the joints, and, most important, effective. In just 12 movements, you'll stretch and strengthen muscles in your arms, shoulders, back, chest, legs, and buns. Do you want firm arms, more toned thighs, a flatter tummy, and slimmer hips? Then this routine is for you.

The *Eat Carbs, Lose Weight* routine requires no equipment. That's right. No dumbbells, no aerobics step, no ball, no bands . . . nothing. Although those pieces of equipment are very effective, I wanted to design a routine that you could do anywhere at any time. Whether you found yourself in a hotel room, in your office at work, or at home with your baby, I wanted you to be able to complete your routine.

Instead of resistance from weights or exercise bands, you'll use your own body weight as resistance for these moves. You always have your body with you, wherever you go. So you'll never have an excuse not to exercise!

This routine is also gentle on your knees, back, and other joints. It includes no bouncy, jerky, or straining motions. That's the beauty of yoga and Pilates. The motions are slow, controlled, and gentle.

To make the routine as efficient as possible, I included moves that strengthen and stretch your muscles simultaneously. The strengthening action will tone, firm, and sculpt muscles in your arms, legs, abdomen, and buns. The stretching action will lengthen your muscles, creating a long, lean appearance. When you stretch, you extend the ends of your muscles, creating space for oxygen to flow more freely. Regular stretching also increases your energy. As you increase flexibility, your body will hold less tension and move more fluidly with less tightness. Also, stretching pumps blood into your muscles and releases tension from them, which generally makes you feel good. This circulation helps to heal your body, patching up any injuries and soothing away aches and pains.

For optimum success, follow these pointers.

Move at your own pace. Some of the movements—such as the pushup and reverse plank—are challenging. For the more challenging moves, I've suggested ways to modify the pose. For example, with the pushup, you might start with your knees on the ground. As you build strength, you may eventually do advanced pushups with your legs extended. For each exercise, I've also specified an amount of time to hold or repeat a movement. You may need to work up to this amount of time. Feel free to take breaks. Do your best, and soon you'll find that you are strong enough to do each movement with perfect technique.

Go in order. The *Eat Carbs, Lose Weight* routine flows from standing to sitting to lying. Each move in the sequence has a certain purpose and benefit. Performing the moves in this order also helps you to ease into the next set of muscles.

Go longer if you have the time. Twelve minutes is the minimum for this routine. If you have more time or want to see faster results, you can do this routine twice a day.

Make exercise a habit. I recommend you complete this routine every day. Make it a habit, just like brushing your teeth. Do it in the morning right after you get out of bed, during the day as a nice energizing break, or even in the evening as a "nightcap." If you've never exercised before, I recommend you do the routine at the same time every day. This will help to make exercise a habit that will last for a lifetime. I like to do it in the morning, right after my walk or cardio workout.

1. TOTAL BODY STRETCH

I love how this stretch makes me feel. It's a wonderful way to warm up your back and sides. I do this stretch whenever I've been working at my desk and need a stretch break. It feels fantastic.

A. Stand with your feet close together. Raise your arms overhead and place your fingers in a temple position, as shown. Inhale as you grow taller from your feet to the top of your head.

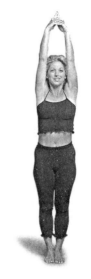

B. Exhale as you reach up and over with your fingertips and bend to the left. Hold for 5 seconds, inhale as you rise to center, and repeat on the other side. Continue alternating sides for 1 minute.

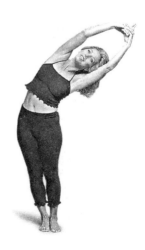

2. WARRIOR II

Similar to a lunge, this incredible thigh-slimming yoga pose will also stretch your legs and hips. If you reach your fingertips away from each other, you will open up the chest and firm your arms as you strengthen your legs and buns.

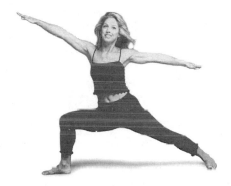

From total body stretch, step out with your right leg, placing your feet about a leg's distance away from each other. Turn out your right foot 90 degrees and slide your left heel back slightly. Place your hands on your hips. Exhale as you bend your right knee until your right thigh is parallel with the floor. Look to your left.

Extend your arms laterally from your shoulders, as shown. Reach your fingertips apart and keep your shoulders low, away from your ears. Hold up to 30 seconds, taking deep breaths, and then repeat on the other side.

3. PUSHUP

Whether you do them on your knees or with your legs extended, pushups help strengthen the chest and upper arms. They'll also get your heart rate up and provide you with a sense of accomplishment. Start with whatever amount you can do— even if it's one or two pushups. Take a break and try again. Once you can repeat the movement for 1 minute, give yourself an enthusiastic pat on the back!

Option 1: On Your Knees

A. From warrior II, bring your feet back together, bend forward from the waist, place your hands on the floor, and extend one leg and then the other. Then lower your knees to the floor.

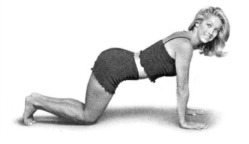

B. With a straight back and tight buns, bend your elbows as you inhale and lower yourself as far as you can toward the floor. Exhale as you straighten your arms and press up to the starting position. Repeat 15 times.

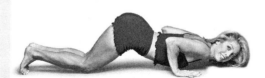

Option 2 (advanced):
With Straight Legs

A. From warrior II, bring your feet back together, bend forward from the waist, place your hands on the floor, and extend one leg and then the other. Make sure your palms are under your collarbones and balance on the balls of your feet, as shown.

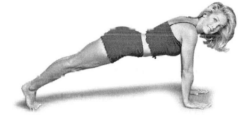

B. With a straight back, slowly bend your elbows as you inhale and lower your chest as close to the floor as you can while still being able to push back up. Exhale and straighten your elbows as you press up. Repeat 15 times.

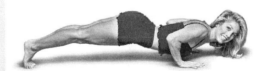

4. LOW HOVER

This is a great ab exercise. You'll firm your upper body as you simultaneously strengthen your midsection. This is a challenging move. Do your best and you'll be rewarded with a tight tummy and firm arms!

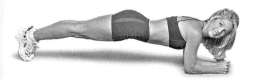

Start on your tummy with your legs extended. Clasp your hands together in front of you. Inhale and then exhale as you lift your legs and torso into the hover, raising your entire torso a few inches off the floor while keeping your elbows in close to your torso. Hold up to 1 minute, taking numerous breaks if needed.

5. TUSH TIGHTENER AND BACK STRENGTHENER

Keep your tummy tight as you extend your arm away from your leg. In addition to helping you to flatten that tummy, this exercise strengthens the muscles that line the spine. The erector muscles need to stay strong for good balance and posture.

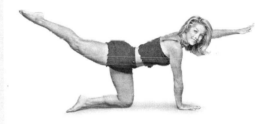

Get on all fours, with your hands flat on the floor under your shoulders and your knees under your hips.

Pulling your abs in, exhale and extend your left arm and right leg until both are parallel to the floor. Hold for 5 seconds as you squeeze your buttocks. Return your loft arm and right leg to the starting posi- tion as you inhale. Then exhale and extend your right arm and left leg. Continue alter- nating up to 1 minute.

6. CRISSCROSS/BICYCLE

Researchers have determined that this is the most effective abdominal exercise you can do. It strengthens your obliques, the abdominal muscles that form your waist, as well as the front of your abdomen.

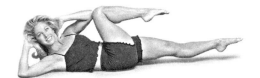

Lie on your back with your head resting back into your fingertips. Your elbows should be open to the sides. Bend your knees, placing your feet flat on the floor. Contract your abs and lift both feet off the floor.

Exhale as you extend your left leg and simultaneously bring your right knee toward your chest. At the same time, rotate your shoulders, bringing your left elbow toward your right knee, as shown. Inhale as you change positions. Once your shoulders almost reach the floor, exhale and repeat the move by extending your right leg and bringing your left knee in toward your chest. Repeat the entire sequence up to 1 minute, aiming for about 25 total repetitions.

7. BRIDGE/THIGH FIRMER

When done correctly, the bridge allows you to firm and stretch multiple muscles at once. In particular, you'll firm your deepest abdominal muscle—the transverse abdominis—as you tuck your tailbone to protect your lower back when it's in an arched position. You'll also stretch your hip flexors and strengthen the backs of your thighs and buttocks.

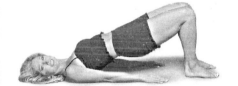

Lie on your back with your knees bent and your feet flat on the floor. Rest your arms at your sides, with your palms down and at about hip level. Take a deep breath.

Exhale as you contract your abs, tuck your tailbone, and curl your hips up, as shown, using your abs to lift your torso. Use your hands for balance, but don't use them to push yourself up. Hold up to 1 minute, taking a break or two if needed. During your break, pull your knees into your chest to stretch your lower back.

8. LOWER TUMMY FIRMER

This wonderful Pilates move will help firm your lower abdomen (below the navel). Try not to let the weight of your legs pull you into the rollover. You want to work those lower abs, not let gravity do the work for you.

A. Lie on your back and rest your arms at your sides. Lift your feet toward the ceiling as you extend your legs, forming a 90-degree angle between your legs and torso. Press your inner thighs and heels together as you rotate your toes slightly outward.

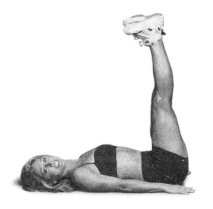

B. With flat, tight abs, exhale and curl your hips toward your ribs, curling up slowly, just one vertebra at a time. Once you cannot curl your lower body any farther, inhale and slowly lower just one vertebra at a time. Repeat lifting and lowering slowly 15 times.

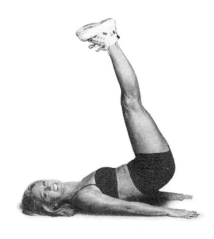

9. SIDE LEG LIFT

This Pilates movement will strengthen and lengthen your legs, especially your outer thighs. You'll also stretch your inner thighs. It's great for your waistline and slimming your hips, too!

Lie on your left side with your legs extended, toes pointed, and your head cradled in your left hand. Rest your right hand on the floor near your chest. Engage and tighten your abs in toward your spine.

With your right leg slightly turned out, inhale as you raise your right leg toward the ceiling, as shown. Hold 2 seconds as you keep your right thigh and legs firm. Lower and repeat 15 times before switching sides.

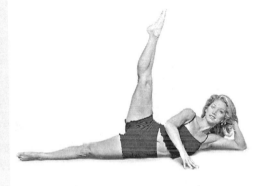

10. REVERSE PLANK

You'll firm your arms, legs, upper back, and buns as you simultaneously stretch your legs and chest. You'll also work the deepest layer of your abdomen as you stabilize your torso. If this move feels too challenging for you, try it with your knees bent, so that your body forms the shape of a table.

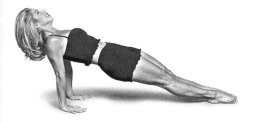

Sit on the floor with your legs extended in front of you and your hands pressed into the floor next to your buttocks. Firm your abs as you exhale and press into your palms, straightening your arms and lifting your hips toward the ceiling, as shown. Your forehead, shoulders, hips, and heels should form a straight line. Make sure your shoulder blades are pushed back and low on your back, so that your chest is open and your neck is long. Imagine that a string is pulling your chest toward the ceiling. Hold up to 30 seconds, taking breaks if needed.

If you take a break, relax for a few seconds by lying on your back with your knees pulled into your chest.

11. DOWN DOG

This quintessential yoga posture will sculpt your shoulders and your arms, strengthen your midback, and stretch your legs, spine, and chest. This is a fantastic stretch that helps to revitalize you.

A. Get on your hands and knees.

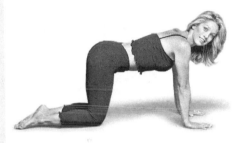

B. Press back through your palms and bring your buttocks close to your heels. Lower both heels toward the floor and extend through both legs, raising your tailbone toward the ceiling, as shown. Widen your shoulder blades and turn the creases of your elbows inward and upward. Gaze at your navel to keep your neck in a neutral position. Hold up to 1 minute, taking breaks if needed.

If you need to take a break, rest in the child's pose by bending your knees and bringing your buttocks toward your heels.

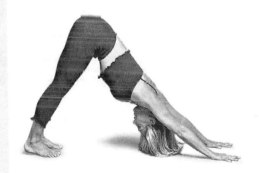

12. HIP STRETCH

This is my favorite yoga stretch. It will relax and lengthen your piriformis muscle, a deep muscle in your buttocks that, when tight, is often responsible for back pain and sciatica. You'll also stretch your outer thighs and hips. If you feel very tight when you try this stretch, place a small pillow under the buttock of your bent leg. This will reduce the angle of the stretch, making it less intense.

A. From down dog, lower your buttocks until you are in a plank position, so a straight line forms from your heels to your head. Bring your left knee forward between your hands, just to the inside of your left wrist, placing your left foot near your right hand.

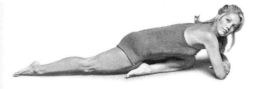

B. Exhale and extend back through your right leg, sinking deeper into the stretch. For an even deeper stretch, extend your arms to the sides, as shown. Hold up to 30 seconds, breathing normally, and then repeat with the other leg.

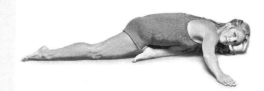

"I Ate Carbs and Lost Weight!"

Name: Susan Jahns

Age: 41

Town: Clermont, Florida

Weight Lost: 12 pounds in 4 weeks

Other Accomplishments: Got the jump start she needed

"I've been through a lot in my life, including a sexual assault, which resulted in a terrible bout of depression and weight gain. My highest weight was 192. About 6 years ago I lost 75 pounds through diet and exercise, but in the past few years I began having the same problems (I entered an abusive relationship), and my weight rose to 180.

"Recently my self-esteem and self-worth came back, but I was having a hard time losing even a pound because of added stress. My oldest daughter relocated to Florida to finish school and to work, and it's been a slow, stressful process.

"The first reason I decided to lose the weight was truly for myself, and the second reason was for my daughter and my son, because I want to be around for them as long as possible. I also have learned that life is truly worth living, no matter how bad things get.

"Stress has always been a major factor in my life, and I've been trying everything I can to reduce it, but I need help. Thanks to Denise for giving me some of the help I needed.

"Over the 28 days I was on *Eat Carbs, Lose Weight*, I lost 12 pounds. I really liked the program because I got to eat real food. The recipes were tasty and not too complicated to make. I still have some additional pounds to lose, but *Eat Carbs, Lose Weight* gave me the jump start I needed to get going."

6

THE SECRETS BEHIND THE *EAT CARBS, LOSE WEIGHT* MEAL PLAN

Find out how to eat cake (and other carbs), lose weight, and stay healthy for life

If you've tried many diets in the past, you've probably heard about those so-called magical ingredients in various foods that help melt away fat. The truth is, there are no miracle foods that rev up the metabolism or melt away fat. Although certain types of foods can certainly aid your fat-burning efforts, the winning formula for weight loss is really very simple: Calories in must be a smaller number than calories out. In other words, you must burn more calories than you eat.

Indeed, all diets work on this important principle. Whether you have tried low carb, low fat, grapefruit, or cabbage soup, all of these diets helped you to lose weight by getting you to eat fewer calories. The *Eat Carbs, Lose Weight* plan is no different. On this plan, you will consume 1,300 calories a day, which, for many of us, totals about 250 to 500 fewer calories than we are currently eating. You'll also burn an additional 50 to 100 calories a day through the *Eat Carbs, Lose Weight* exercise plan, plus another 300 to 400 on your cardio-walk days. End result: You will burn more calories than you eat and lose up to 2 pounds a week.

You might be thinking, "If losing weight and keeping it off were only as simple as eating less and exercising more, why isn't everyone doing it? Why isn't everyone trim? How come most diets don't work?"

Aah, now we get to the science of weight loss. Whereas most diets succeed in helping people to lose weight, few achieve the most important challenge of all: helping people to keep off the weight. To keep off the weight, you must adopt an eating plan that you can stick with for a lifetime. Can you eat cabbage soup every day for the rest of your life? How about grapefruit? What about lots of protein and hardly any carbs? For most of us, the answers to those questions are *no, no,* and *no.*

This is what sets the *Eat Carbs, Lose Weight* menu plan apart from diets you may have tried in the past. Not only will you be eating fewer calories than you burn, you will be eating in a way that you can stick with long term. Because you will eat a variety of foods every day, your meals will never become monotonous. Unlike many diets that claim to help you lose weight with so-called magical ingredients, you'll never look at your breakfast, lunch, or dinner plate and think to yourself, "Oh, not *this* again."

In addition to a variety of foods, you will also eat reasonable portions of some savory and downright delectable foods. The Orange-Scented Cornmeal Cake with Fresh Berries, Peach Melba, and other sweet desserts on this plan will have your taste buds in seventh heaven. On this plan, you'll never yearn to eat a banned food, because there are no banned foods. You'll enjoy every meal on this plan, and this is possibly the most important reason why the *Eat Carbs, Lose Weight* plan works long term. When you love what you eat, you'll more easily find the motivation to stick with your eating plan for life.

On this plan, you'll eat a healthful balance of nutrient-dense, low-refined-carb foods. You'll consume plenty of fiber and phytonutrients from fruits, vegetables, and whole grains. You'll also eat satisfying amounts of lean protein from chicken, fish, turkey, and even pork and beef. And, yes, you'll also consume some fat, enough to add that all-important delicious taste and mouthwatering texture to your meals. You'll tap into your own body's natural instincts about nutrition to help you lose weight and keep it off in the following ways.

⬦ You'll preserve fat-burning muscle mass as you lose weight. This will keep your energy levels up for your exercise plan as well as maintain your metabolism.

⬦ You'll eat foods that will help allow you to feel fuller on fewer calories.

⬦ You'll eat in a way that helps optimize your mood and energy levels. This will not only give you more motivation to move but also help reduce unplanned snacking and cravings.

So how does the *Eat Carbs, Lose Weight* plan accomplish all of this? It all starts with the right breakdown of carbohydrates, proteins, and fats.

THE 50–25–25 PLAN

If you've tried many diets, you've probably eaten all sorts of combinations of carbohydrates, proteins, and fats. During the 1980s and 1990s, for example, you may have kept your fat calories as low as 10 percent and your carbohydrate calories as high as 70 percent of your total calories for the day. If you've tried low-carb diets, then you've also done the opposite, holding your carbohydrate calories to just 5 or 10 percent of your daily total and making up the rest with protein and fat.

So why do nutritionist Amy Campbell and I feel that 50 percent of calories from carbs and 25 percent of calories each from protein and fat provide the best macronutrient breakdown for weight loss?

Let's first talk about carbs. When you go below 50 percent, you don't provide your body with enough dietary carbohydrate to fuel your brain and muscles. If you remember from chapter 2, your brain needs a *minimum* of 130 grams of carbohydrates a day to function optimally. If you dip under that 50 percent threshold, you might feel dull, notice frequent headaches, and suddenly can't remember your coworker's name or where you placed your car keys. If you exercise, going under 50 percent does not allow your body to optimally store carbohydrate in your muscles. Because your muscles use this fuel during exercise, you will feel fatigued during your workout sessions, especially when you exercise 2 days in a row.

On the other hand, going above 50 percent may fuel you with *too many* carbs. Although some enviable people can certainly eat more carbohydrate and remain slim and trim, most people cannot. If you are overweight, your body does not process blood sugar as efficiently as the body of someone who is at a normal weight. Eating too many carbs will flood your system with too much sugar at once, spiking insulin levels and causing premature hunger and fatigue. Although it may seem counterintuitive, going above 50 percent may also cause you to crave and binge on sweets. When you consume more than 50 percent of your calories from carbs, that means you must consume less protein and fat. As you'll soon learn, going below 25 percent of calories for either of these macronutrients can result in hunger, overeating, and carbohydrate cravings.

So, with that said, let's talk about fat. Despite popular belief, fat actually performs a number of important functions in the human body. It helps to form vital hormones and give your skin a healthy glow. Without some fat, your body would not be able to absorb some vitamins, such as A, D, E, and K. When you eat the right amounts of the right types of fat, you lose weight and improve your health. On the other hand, eating the wrong amount—either too little or too much—can spell dietary disaster.

First, the evils of eating too little: During the nonfat years, many people tried to nearly eliminate fat from their diets. Well, guess what? Most of them ended up *gaining* weight, not losing it. Why? You must consume reasonable amounts of fat in order to find the motivation to stick to your meal plan. Most important, fat helps to slow digestion. Research shows that high-carbohydrate, nonfat foods (such as fat-free muffins) do not fill people up and tend to cause premature hunger and cravings. On the other hand, eating muffins that contain a little fat will cause you to feel more satisfied—for many hours to come.

Second, fat adds a delicious taste and texture to foods. Think of the creaminess of ice cream, the moistness of chocolate cake, and the crispiness of a cookie. Nonfat versions of those foods just don't compare with the real thing. Deny yourself the occasional indulgence, and your desire for these foods will build until you can no longer stand it. Instead of eating a few spoonfuls of ice cream, you'll end up eating the entire half gallon!

Certain types of fat—such as the omega-3 fatty acids found in salmon and flaxseed products and the omega-6 fatty acids found in olive and canola oils—are also good for your health. Omega-3 fatty acids in particular have been shown to lift depression and boost mood. Eating the right amounts of these fats may help you to reduce cravings for unhealthy carbs if you tend to turn to them when you feel depressed.

Omega-3 and omega-6 fats have also been shown to reduce heart disease and cancer risk. A study published in the *American Journal of Clinical Nutrition* found that the human body can only absorb the carotenoids (a type of phytonutrient) from a salad if the salad contains some fat in the dressing. In fact, the greatest amount of carotenoids were absorbed in the intestines when participants ate salads with full-fat dressing, versus reduced-fat dressing.

That said, you don't want to go overboard. Fat does contain 9 calories per gram, compared with just 4 calories per gram of protein or carbohydrate. Going much above 25 percent of your total calories allows those excess calories to add up. In short, too much of a good thing can add up to too much fat on your tummy and thighs.

The same logic applies to protein. Like fat, protein helps to slow digestion and ease the entrance of sugar into the bloodstream. This helps you feel satisfied on fewer calories. Also, research shows that eating 25 percent of calories from protein can help dieters maintain muscle mass as they lose weight. This is critical, because, as I've mentioned before, your muscle mass is one of the only aspects of your metabolism within your control. Every pound of muscle burns 35 to 50 calories a day just to maintain itself—and countless more calories every time it powers movement. When you lose weight, you want the weight to come from your fat stores—and not from your muscle. Keeping your protein consumption to roughly 25 percent of your total calories helps you to do just that. (Also, including regular muscle-sculpting exercise is essential to maintaining muscle mass, which is why I recommend a daily 12-minute routine.)

As an added bonus, eating this amount of protein will probably boost your energy level as well, especially if you've been skimping on protein in the past. Certain amino acids in protein foods increase amounts of the amino acid tyrosine in the brain. This amino acid is used to manufacture the neurotransmitters dopamine, norepinephrine, and epinephrine. When levels of these neurotransmitters are optimal, you feel more physically and mentally alert.

Although protein is certainly important to weight loss, going above 25 percent—as many low-carb diets recommend—may be hazardous to your health. Diets that contain more than 30 percent of their calories from protein may increase the risk of dehydration (which, in turn, makes you feel fatigued), kidney stones, gallstones, and possibly even bone loss.

THREE MEALS AND TWO SNACKS

On this plan, you'll spread your 1,300 daily calories over three meals and two snacks. This means you'll have something to eat every 3 to 4 hours, providing both the psychological and the nutritional motivation you need to stick to the plan.

Psychologically, it's much easier to avoid unplanned, unhealthy snacking (and overeating) when you know your next meal or snack is only 3 hours away. Planning snacks into your day also helps ensure you eat snacks that help promote weight loss rather than snacks that promote weight gain. For example, have you ever found yourself raiding the fridge after work because you were so hungry you couldn't wait until dinner? What did you eat? Chances are, it wasn't brussels sprouts!

When you plan your snacks into your day, you avoid this dangerous bingeing. By eating smaller amounts of carbohydrates more frequently, you'll more easily be able to stabilize your blood sugar. This helps you avoid those peaks and valleys in your energy levels that can lead to cravings, overeating, and the midafternoon slump. Your snacks also allow you to eat something at precisely the time a craving is likely to hit—helping you to avoid raiding the fridge or the vending machine at work.

Best of all, your snacks aren't just an afterthought—they're delicious mini-meals of varied tastes and textures, rich in satisfying carbs. On the *Eat Carbs, Lose Weight* plan, you'll be snacking on graham crackers smeared with peanut butter, frozen grapes, celery dipped in hummus, frozen papaya chunks, peanuts, almonds, fresh fruit, Parmesan-covered popcorn, baked apples, and banana bread covered with creamy butter, among many other snacks. Your snacks will contain some protein or fiber—or both—to stabilize blood sugar levels and reduce your appetite. All of the snacks are designed to give you the staying power you need to make it to your next meal. It's all balanced.

THE RIGHT CARBS

In addition to providing the right balance of carbohydrates for weight loss, the *Eat Carbs, Lose Weight* plan optimizes your consumption of blood sugar–friendly carbs. Better still, it minimizes your consumption of the types of carbs that are digested quickly and trigger cravings for yet more carbs.

From salads and stir-fries to smoothies and sandwiches, you'll be eating plenty of fresh fruit, vegetables, legumes, and whole grains. All of these foods are high in fiber, which slows the transport of sugar into the bloodstream. Fiber also helps you to feel fuller sooner when you eat, helping to keep you from overeating.

Some of the carbs on this plan, however, I've included simply because they are, well, delicious. Life's too short to forgo the occasional bite of cheesecake or delectable serving of Pears Baked in Rum Cream Sauce. You'll find all of these carbohydrate foods—

Proactive Snacking

To make sure you stick to the food plan and eat the right types of snacks, each evening look over your meal plan for the following day. Make sure you have your ingredients on hand. Measure out your snacks and place them in plastic bags. Remember, you eat what you see, so allow yourself to see *only* what you plan to eat.

and more—on the meal plan. Yes, they are high in sugar. Yes, they are low in fiber. And, yes, they are all delicious. That's the point!

You could follow the healthiest meal plan in the world—one that strictly included the best carbohydrates, proteins, and fats. You would lose weight. But could you stick to a plan like that long term? I know I couldn't. As I've mentioned before, the *Eat Carbs, Lose Weight* plan reflects how I really eat. The plan wouldn't be true to life—or realistic—if it didn't include some indulgent treats!

Including some sweets in your meal plan will aid your weight-loss efforts—not detract from them. Each day, your 1,300 calories will include your yummy desserts. So, despite eating such satisfying desserts, you'll be eating fewer calories than your body needs, which will spur weight loss. Also, the other healthy foods that make up the bulk of the food plan will help to drive down your appetite and fill in any nutritional gaps. So go ahead and enjoy that piece of cheesecake on Day 28 or the pears on Day 24. You deserve them.

THE RIGHT FATS

Although all types of fat contain 9 calories per gram—making them equally as fattening—not all fats affect your health the same way. And although your body can manufacture 18 of the 20 fatty acids needed for good health, you must consume two of them through your diet: omega-3 and omega-6 fatty acids.

The monounsaturated omega-6 fatty acids found in olive and canola oils help to reduce heart disease and may prevent certain types of cancer, such as breast and colon cancer. Various studies show that this type of fat can increase LDL particle size, rendering this unhealthy type of cholesterol less likely to clog your arteries. This fat also has been shown to reduce blood pressure.

The omega-3 fatty acids found in fish and flaxseeds are equally beneficial at boosting heart health. This important type of fat may also help lift depression, which, in turn, can help reduce food cravings and overeating.

To optimize your consumption of the healthful omega-3 and omega-6 fatty acids, the *Eat Carbs, Lose Weight* plan includes added fats from olive and canola oils. You will be using those oils for cooking and on top of your salads. You'll also be eating plenty of fish and some ground flaxseeds and walnuts for those wonderful omega-3 fatty acids.

You won't, however, be eating much saturated fat or many trans fatty acids, both of which have been implicated in heart disease. Found in animal products such as red meat and cheese, saturated fats increase levels of blood cholesterol. This is why you will be consuming lean protein foods such as steak tenderloin, pork tenderloin, and chicken breast.

Trans fatty acids, also called partially hydrogenated oils, may be even worse for your health than saturated fats. Developed during the 1930s, these synthetic fats are solid at room temperature. Created in large refinery-like factories, trans fats are made from otherwise healthful vegetable oils. To make these oils solid at room temperature, manufacturers bubble hydrogen gas through them at 250° to 400°F. This "hydrogenates" the fat, hardening it. Found in everything from crackers and cinnamon buns to fried foods and margarine, trans fats extend the shelf life of many foods and protect against rancidity. As with saturated fats, they also add a certain texture to baked goods. For example, you can thank trans fats for the flakiness of store-bought piecrust.

Although manufacturers once claimed that these fats were healthier than saturated fats (promoting margarine over butter, for example), research has found the opposite to be true. Studies show that consumption of trans fats increases levels of unhealthy LDL cholesterol and decreases levels of healthy HDL cholesterol. Researchers at Harvard estimate that consumption of these fats results in 30,000 to 100,000 premature cardiac deaths each year. One German study has even found that a high intake of margarine (which contains trans fats) increased the risk of asthma in adults.

I try to eat as little of this type of fat as possible, which is why Amy and I worked hard to nearly eliminate it from the meal plan. Because this fat occurs naturally in some foods—such as dairy products and meat—you will never get your trans fat consumption down to zero (that is, unless you are a vegetarian). Although I'm not suggesting you forgo meat and cheese, I do strongly recommend nearly eliminating any additional trans

"I Ate Carbs and Lost Weight!"

Name: Donna Yates
Age: 48
Town: Longmont, Colorado
Weight Lost: 11 pounds in 4 weeks
Other Accomplishments: Lost 1½ inches from her waist and hips

"I always felt trapped in an overweight body. I was a chubby baby, and as a teenager, I always thought I was overweight even though I probably wasn't. A couple of years ago, it finally dawned on me that I was not fat then but I certainly have grown into the image I always had of myself. Over the years, my weight slowly rose, partially due to a busy life as an administrative assistant at a local hospital and a stepmother to three boys. Eventually, I found myself 80 pounds overweight.

"To lose the unwanted pounds, I tried myriad diets, from the pineapple diet to the Cambridge diet to low-carb diets. I lost 35 pounds on Atkins in about 3 months, but it was difficult to stick to, and I was concerned that it wasn't all that healthy.

"And after reading articles about the potentially harmful effects of low-carb diets, I was looking for a healthy alternative and a diet that I could make a way of life. *Eat Carbs, Lose Weight* has turned out to be exactly what I needed. "After just 28 days on Denise's healthy, good carb plan, I lost 11 pounds and 1½ inches from my waist and hips.

"I am really pleased with my results. I definitely have more energy than I did before. It's easier to get out of bed in the morning and get my exercises done before I make breakfast, and I don't feel worn out by midafternoon. My clothes are looser on me than they have been in a while, and I've been able to dig out and wear some things I haven't been able to get into in a long time. And my husband, of course, noticed my weight loss.

"I also really enjoy the food. The recipes are very flavorful, and the cravings that helped drive my weight up in the first place have disappeared—I think the variety of good foods included in the diet have helped with that. I plan to stick with *Eat Carbs, Lose Weight* until I reach my goal weight loss of 80 pounds and beyond."

Donna's advice: "I would advise other women on the diet to get their families involved. My husband was pretty supportive and was willing to try most of the foods I prepared. It's helpful to have someone to support you while you make a lifestyle change."

fats. The *Eat Carbs, Lose Weight* plan does just that. Although this fat lurks in nearly all processed foods, we've done the homework to find brands of crackers and breakfast cereals that don't contain it or are as low in this fat as possible.

THE RIGHT PROTEIN FOODS

When you see some of the protein choices on the *Eat Carbs, Lose Weight* plan, you might wonder if you have died and gone to heaven. You'll be eating steak, ham, and pork, among many other protein foods. But the difference is, this won't be *all* that you're eating.

I've always believed that you can enjoy the most delicious protein foods without all of the artery-clogging saturated fat—and the *Eat Carbs, Lose Weight* meal plan proves it. Yes, you'll eat red meat from time to time, but it will be *lean* red meat. For example, you'll be eating steak tenderloin, which is one of the leanest cuts of steak around. Similarly, you'll have pork tenderloin and extra-lean ham.

In addition to lean sources of red meat, the plan includes skinless chicken breast and thighs, which are also low in saturated fat. You'll also be eating plenty of fish. Naturally low in saturated fat and calories, fish is truly one of nature's best weight-loss foods. And contrary to some people's perceptions, it's also incredibly easy to cook, making it the ideal food for on-the-go dieters.

The plan even calls for some eggs, which you'll often be eating hard boiled or poached. These are the healthiest ways to cook eggs, because these cooking methods require no butter or oil. Hard-boiled eggs offer a perfect snack, as they contain only 70 calories and are easy to make and pack. Just hard-boil a dozen at the beginning of the week and take one to work with you for a great low-calorie, lean-protein snack.

Finally, on the *Eat Carbs, Lose Weight* plan, you'll consume peanuts, almonds, and walnuts. These delicious snacks will help give you the staying power you need to make it from one meal to another. With their crunchy, buttery consistency, they also satisfy your taste buds, which can fuel your motivation to make better food choices all day long. For example, a study done at Loma Linda University in California found that participants spontaneously consumed more fiber and vegetables and fewer trans fatty acids and simple sugars once they added more nuts to their diet.

Nuts themselves are some of nature's most potent power foods. In a study completed at Pennington Biomedical Research Center at Louisiana State University in Baton

The Right Supplements

On the *Eat Carbs, Lose Weight* plan, you will maximize your consumption of nutrient-packed foods. Every bite of fruits, vegetables, and whole grains has numerous health benefits. Still, in today's stressful world of processed foods and sometimes less-than-optimally-grown produce, you should take a multivitamin/mineral to fill in any possible dietary gaps, just to be safe. Follow these tips when choosing a multivitamin/mineral.

✧ Look for the U.S. Pharmacopoeia symbol (USP). This means the vitamin meets criteria for quality assurance and has been tested under strict laboratory conditions.

✧ Make sure the supplement contains 100 percent of the DV (Daily Value) for thiamin (B_1), riboflavin (D_2), niacin (B_3), B_6, B_{12}, folic acid, and vitamin D.

✧ Choose a supplement that contains at least 20 micrograms of vitamin K.

✧ Choose a supplement that contains up to 100 percent of the following: chromium, copper, iodine, selenium, and zinc.

◊ Buy no vitamin that contains more than 100 percent of the DV for vitamin A. Because this vitamin is fat soluble, too much of it can easily become toxic. Make sure that at least 40 percent of vitamin A in the multi comes from beta-carotene.

✧ If you are a woman who is menstruating, choose a multi that contains 100 percent of the DV for iron. If you are postmenopausal or male, choose a multi that either contains no iron or has less than 45 percent of the DV for iron.

✧ If you have premenstrual syndrome, opting for a supplement with the following amounts of the following nutrients may help alleviate irritability, fluid retention, joint aches, breast tenderness, anxiety, depression, and fatigue: B_6 (100 micrograms), vitamin C (1,000 milligrams), vitamin E (400 international units), and magnesium (300 milligrams).

In addition to your multi, please consider taking a calcium supplement. Ladies, after menopause, take one that contains 1,200 to 1,500 milligrams of calcium a day. If you are menstruating, take one that contains about 1,000 to 1,200 milligrams. If you are a man older than age 65, look for one with 1,200 to 1,500 milligrams. If you are a man younger than age 65, take 1,000 milligrams.

Rouge, 20 people with diabetes who added almonds to their diets lowered their bad LDL cholesterol as much as 29 percent. Another study completed at Loma Linda University found similar results: that daily almond consumption helped to lower levels of the unhealthy LDL cholesterol and increase levels of the healthy HDL cholesterol.

THE RIGHT DECADENCE

If you skim through the menus, you'll notice a couple of food options that seem anything but diet foods. You'll find some red meat, some cheese, and some scrumptious desserts such as Orange Cheesecake with Glazed Blueberries and Gingered Pumpkin Pudding. What are these foods doing on a menu in a weight-loss book?

As I've said before, you need moderation, variety, and balance so that you can eat healthily for life in order to keep off the weight. If you make your meal options too restrictive, you won't be able to stick to your plan. I've always believed that it's much better to have a little bit of decadence every day than a lot of decadence every once in a while.

Yes, you want to eat smart carbs, lean proteins, and the right fats—most of the time. But we're all human, and we love our food, so we need treats, too. For weight loss to last long term, you must be able to consume foods that make your mouth water and give you a sense of comfort and satisfaction.

Speaking of long-term weight loss, you can keep the weight off only if you know how to eat long term. The *Eat Carbs, Lose Weight* plan includes 4 weeks of menus. That doesn't mean you'll revert to eating junk after this plan is over! Many of the benefits we've talked about—reduced blood pressure, improved mood, better control of blood sugar, not to mention lasting weight loss—are best enjoyed long term. You finally have an eating plan you can savor and really imagine staying on for life—so stick with it! These 4 weeks are just the beginning of a whole new approach to healthy, energizing, life-enhancing nutrition. You deserve to feel this good *forever.*

7

EAT CARBS FOR LIFE

Reach your goal and keep off the weight

I loved the movie *Groundhog Day*, the one where Bill Murray repeats the same day over and over again. No matter how much he accomplished during the day, he always went to bed at night and then reawakened to live Groundhog Day all over again. I remember laughing at that movie, yet I know that for many women trying to lose weight, the theme of the movie resonates poignantly. Many of my fans tell me that with each new diet, they manage to lose some weight only to eventually reawake with the same layers of fat on their belly, thighs, and buns. For them, weight loss has become a frustrating cycle of lose, regain, lose, and regain.

If this sounds all too familiar to you, I have wonderful news. I'm here to tell you that you *can* break this frustrating cycle. You *can* lose weight and keep it off. Although I've heard from many people who are stuck in the lose-regain cycle, I also have heard from thousands who have broken the cycle and lost the weight for good! These fans e-mail and write to me, telling me about their wonderful success. You may even know some of them, because I like to feature them on my morning television show or on my Web site, DeniseAustin.com!

Over the years, these fans have shared with me their secrets for keeping off the weight. In addition to what they tell me, I've also closely followed the results of a long-term study about what it takes not only to lose weight but also to keep it off for good.

In this study, researchers have begun to track "successful maintainers." Thousands of men and women have shared their secrets of success with researchers at the University of Colorado and the University of Pittsburgh, who since 1993 have kept a database of successful maintainers, people who have lost 30 or more pounds and kept it off for more than a year. The researchers push no particular diet or weight-loss plan. Rather, they ask successful maintainers around the country to log on to their National Weight Control Registry and answer some questions about how they lost weight and, more important, kept it off. So far, more than 4,000 women and men have done just that.

We have much to learn from these 4,000 people. They have lost stunning amounts of weight, with the average Weight Control Registry participant reporting a 60-pound loss. They've also kept it off long term—an average of 5 years or more. Yet, losing weight and keeping it off didn't come naturally for these folks. Many had unsuccessfully tried to lose weight many times before they stumbled upon a plan that worked for them. Two-thirds of them had struggled with their weight since childhood, and 60 percent came from overweight families. Even though genetics were working against them, they triumphed—and you can, too!

Over the years, these researchers have looked at the answers the thousands of successful maintainers have submitted to the National Weight Control Registry and searched for common themes. Although not all of the participants lost weight the same way, nearly all of them used a few simple yet crucial tactics to keep the weight off long term.

I will share these successful tactics with you, along with the tactics of my most successful fans, so you can use them to keep off the weight you lose on the *Eat Carbs, Lose Weight* plan. Before you can maintain your weight loss, however, you must reach your goal weight. So, let's first take a look at how you will do just that.

CHOOSING YOUR GOAL WEIGHT

Before you can start your *Eat Carbs, Lose Weight* journey, you must first pick your destination: your goal weight. Arriving at that important number depends on why you want to lose the weight. If you want to improve your health—lower your blood pressure, improve your blood sugar levels, or lower your blood cholesterol—you probably need to lose much less weight than you think. Studies have shown time and time again that you need lose only 7 to 10 percent of your weight to dramatically improve your health. That means, if you weigh 200 pounds, you need to lose only 20 pounds. If you weigh 150 pounds, you need to lose only 15 pounds.

Of course, many of us want to lose weight for additional reasons. Perhaps you want to fit back into your prepregnancy wardrobe or pare down those love handles that suddenly appeared after age 40. Whatever your reasons, try to be as realistic as possible. Choose a goal weight that you've actually seen on your scale at some point in your adult life. Resist the urge to choose a number on the scale that's *lower* than any number you've seen since the age of 21. Also, pick a weight that you think you can maintain. For example, you might be able to get down to 120 pounds to fit into a bathing suit, but will you be able to remain at that weight once the summer ends?

I recommend you choose your goal based on your current weight, height, and waist measurements. So step on the scale first thing in the morning and record your weight. Losing about 10 percent of your weight in 6 months (20 pounds for someone who weighs 200 pounds) is a great weight-loss pace. Aim to lose about 2 pounds a week.

In addition to picking a goal weight, choose a goal waist measurement. Although excess hip and thigh fat may annoy you, it's the excess abdominal fat that can literally kill you. Research shows that excess fat in the abdomen raises your risk for many diseases, including heart disease, diabetes, high blood pressure, and stroke. Place the measuring tape snugly around your waist. This is your baseline measurement. Make it your goal to bring your waist measurement below 35 inches if you are a woman and below 40 inches if you are a man. For fun, you can also take your hip and thigh measurements. Every 4 weeks, take your measurements again. As you see the numbers drop, you'll increase your motivation to stick with the *Eat Carbs, Lose Weight* plan.

Of course, I think the best indicator of your success has nothing to do with the scale or even your measurements. Go by how your clothes fit. Not long after starting the program, you'll notice that you no longer have to leave your top pants button undone. Not long after that, you'll be able to comfortably tuck in your shirts. Then, you'll eventually need to tighten your belt to keep your pants up. Before you know it, you'll need to go shopping because you've dropped a whole dress size. Now that's true success!

HOW TO REACH YOUR GOAL

If you have flipped ahead in the book, you may have noticed that the *Eat Carbs, Lose Weight* meal plan includes 28 days of menus and recipes. Does this mean you will reach your goal weight within 28 days? For some of you, the answer is yes. For others, the answer is no.

You will lose up to 2 pounds a week on the *Eat Carbs, Lose Weight* plan. After 28 days on the plan, that comes to 8 pounds. (Please note: If you do additional exercise, you may lose weight a little more quickly.) This rate of weight loss ensures that you lose weight where you want to—from your fat stores—and not from where you don't—your muscle tissue. Although 8 pounds may not sound as stunning as the results some fad diets promise, this modest, steady weight loss sets you up for long-term success. You'll keep your metabolism running strong and prevent the hunger and deprivation that lead to cheating and bingeing. You won't feel faint, or desperate, or cheated out of life's delicious pleasures. Instead, you'll be able to stick to the plan for life—and that's the *only* way to keep off the weight.

In fact, in a recent study published in the journal *Appetite,* researchers in the United Kingdom determined that the severe calorie restriction associated with rapid weight loss of more than 2 pounds a week contributed to weight regain in *every single case.* In another study published in the *International Journal of Sports Medicine,* dieters who cut more than 750 calories out of their daily diets in order to lose weight rapidly ended up losing the majority of their weight—61 percent of it—from their muscle stores! Losing muscle in this way slows your metabolism and sets you up for regaining the weight you lost! Remember, muscle is your metabolic furnace. It helps you burn calories even while you sleep.

"I Ate Carbs and Lost Weight!"

Name: Brenda Smallwood

Age: 41

Town: New Orleans, Louisiana

Weight Lost: 9 pounds in 4 weeks

Other Accomplishments: Lost 6½ inches and found more time to pamper herself

"I struggled with my weight as a child, but in my twenties I finally found the right combination of diet and exercise—including Denise Austin workouts and daily walking—that kept me fit and trim. But then in my midthirties I hit a roadblock: I was diagnosed with cervical and uterine cancer. My initial prognosis was grim, and I turned to ice cream for comfort.

"Luckily, two surgeries later, I was cancer-free—but the medication used for treatment, the months of inactivity following the surgeries, and the fact that I was suddenly in full-blown menopause left me 60 pounds overweight.

"To combat the weight gain, I tried Weight Watchers, Atkins, Sugar Busters, Dr. Phil's book, fasting—you name it. But nothing seemed to work.

"Then I heard about *Eat Carbs, Lose Weight*. The plan sounded nutritional and healthful, and based on my past experience with Denise, I trusted that anything she was a part of would yield results . . . and I was right.

"It didn't take long for my family and coworkers to see a difference in my appearance. I got comments like 'Are you losing weight?' and 'Did you change your skin-care regimen? You're absolutely glowing!'

"I really enjoy the variety of foods in the program, and my energy level is the highest it's been in the 3 years since I completed my cancer treatment. My unhealthy cravings are gone—now I crave fruits and vegetables! And I also found more time for a little pampering, like a soak in the tub or a walk with my dog. Everything seemed to fall into place.

"I am excited and encouraged by my results: 9 pounds and 6½ inches lost so far. I plan to stick with the program so I can continue to lose weight and become healthier in the process. I'm so happy to be a part of *Eat Carbs, Lose Weight!*"

Brenda's advice: "Make small changes in your schedule to enable yourself to make more time to focus on yourself and the plan. You will have more energy, you will sleep better, your skin will glow from within, and it will feel almost effortless!"

So promise me—and yourself—right now that you will find the patience and you will recognize the wisdom of this pace of weight loss and how effective it is over the long term. If you have only 4 to 8 pounds to lose, the long term for you comes to 14 to 28 days. Once you've cycled through the plan one time, you'll probably be ready to move on to the *Eat Carbs, Lose Weight* maintenance plan. If, however, you want to lose 20, 30, 40, or more pounds, you'll stick with the weight-loss segment of the *Eat Carbs, Lose Weight* plan for a bit longer. In that case, you'll tackle the plan in two phases. But this is the plan I live with every day because it works. It's for a lifetime.

Phase 1: Day 1 to Day 28

During your first 28 days on the plan, I suggest you follow each meal plan exactly as described. This will encourage you to try every recipe at least once. It will also help you to establish some new habits, such as eating breakfast every day and eating meals and snacks at regular intervals. Sticking to the plan verbatim will help you to lose your first 4 to 8 pounds while on autopilot. You'll have no decisions to make, no calories to count, no food lists to consult. I've done the homework for you. You'll simply follow each day as it's presented to you.

That said, allow yourself the flexibility you need to stay successful on the plan. If you see a meal or food presented on the plan that you know you don't like, can't find in the grocery store, are allergic to, or know in your heart of hearts you simply don't have the time or motivation to prepare, go ahead and swap out that day of the plan for another that is more palatable to you!

During this phase, measure out each ingredient, meal, and snack as suggested by the menus. Then, take a good hard look at each meal before you actually eat it. This will help you to mentally be able to recognize accurate food portions. Eventually, you will no longer need your measuring cups and spoons. You'll be able to dish up the right portions automatically.

I personally think phase 1 is the most exciting phase of the journey. You'll no doubt taste some foods and food combinations for the first time. You may never before have considered snacking on an apple with walnuts or frozen grapes along with string cheese. Think of each day—and each meal and snack—as a new weight-loss adventure. You'll get to try new recipes and cooking techniques. You never know: During phase 1, you may try a new recipe that becomes an instant favorite—for you and your entire family!

Phase 2: Day 29 and Beyond

Once you've completed the first 28 days of the meal plan, you'll turn once again to Day 1 and continue to cycle through the plan from Day 1 to Day 28 until you reach your goal. Unlike phase 1 of the plan, however, you can now take some liberties and personalize the plan to your individual likes and lifestyle. In other words, you're not going to continually repeat this exact meal plan for the rest of your life. I'll teach you how to incorporate your favorite foods and recipes into the *Eat Carbs, Lose Weight* lifestyle. You'll be able to go out to eat, navigate an opulent holiday party, even tackle a meal at your mother-in-law's house, all while staying on the plan.

To stick to a weight-loss plan long term—that is, for as long as it takes to reach your goal—you must include foods you love and follow a plan that fits seamlessly into your lifestyle. The foods and meals included on the meal plan are all my personal favorites. I think every meal and snack from Day 1 to Day 28 is simply delicious. That said, I'm a realist. I know not all of you will agree!

The best meal plan for you is packed with all of the foods you love and none of the foods you don't like. There are no one-size-fits-all meal plans out there—including the one in this book. Indeed, the best plan for you is different than the best plan for another woman. You might be an on-the-go person who doesn't like to cook, for example, whereas someone else may love cooking intricate gourmet meals. You might love chicken and dislike fish, whereas someone else might be the opposite—loves fish but does not like chicken.

To personalize your plan, follow these pointers.

Mix and match. Feel free to mix and match various meals from the plan, choosing the ones you liked the most. For example, if you loved the breakfast smoothie but weren't so hot about eating a muffin in the morning, feel free to substitute the smoothie for the muffin. Similarly, you can mix and match different snack, lunch, and dinner options, as long as you keep the makeup of each individual meal intact. In other words, you can substitute the lunch of a multigrain sandwich on Day 3 for the Shrimp and Avocados with Chiles and Lime lunch on Day 10 as long as you eat your sandwich along with a glass of fat-free milk, as suggested on the menu for that day. Have fun experimenting and interchanging all of the meals, but think of each as a unit—all side dishes, drinks, and so on travel with that meal. In this way, you'll be sure to consume balanced portions of carbohydrates, protein, and fat and keep it healthy.

For those of you who are on the go and don't have much time to spend in the kitchen, this means you can opt for the easiest breakfast, lunch, and dinner meals as well. Choose the cereal with berries over the Coffee-Chocolate Waffles, for example. For lunch, choose from any of the many types of sandwiches, such as the turkey wrap or tuna sandwich. For dinner, you can't beat the ease of beans and rice, broiled fish or meat, or a stir-fry.

Substitute your favorites. In addition to mixing and matching various breakfast, lunch, and dinner options, you can also substitute some ingredients for others. For any recipe, you can substitute any lean protein food for another lean protein food listed in a recipe. For example, you can substitute the same amount of chicken for the same amount of fish in a recipe. (You must, however, stick with lean protein choices. You can't substitute fatty prime rib for skinless chicken breast.) Similarly, if you love ice cream but are not so hot about cheesecake or pudding, substitute a controlled serving of ice cream for those desserts. If you have a shellfish allergy, as I do, you can opt for another type of fish or even for chicken or beef. We've even developed a chart that will help you make smart substitutions. (See "The *Eat Carbs, Lose Weight* Substitution Rules," on pages 122 and 123.)

Go frozen. When you are feeling rushed and don't have time to prepare lunch or dinner, opt for a frozen dinner. This will help you to stay on track long term, allowing the *Eat Carbs, Lose Weight* plan to conveniently fit into your busy lifestyle. Choose frozen entrées with no more than 300 calories, 12 grams of total fat, 5 grams of saturated fat, and 800 milligrams of sodium. (Hold yourself to 600 milligrams of sodium if you have high blood pressure.) Make sure that your dinner offers 15 to 20 grams of protein as well. Examine the Nutrition Facts label of your frozen dinner carefully. Some entrées include two servings rather than just one. At first glance, you might assume that your burrito grande contains only 300 calories. A closer look might reveal that the 300 calories refers to *half* a burrito and not the whole thing! Round out your dinner with steamed veggies or a salad, along with fruit for dessert.

Follow the formula. For those of you who prefer more freedom and feel tied down by a meal plan, you can certainly design your own *Eat Carbs, Lose Weight* meals. You need only stick to the following formula. Each meal should include roughly:

✧ 45 grams of carbohydrate

✧ 3 to 4 ounces of protein

✧ One to two servings of fat

For your snacks, hold yourself to:

✧ 15 to 20 grams of carbohydrate

✧ Approximately 60 to 80 calories

✧ A bit of fat and protein (It's okay—in fact, preferable—to add a small, healthful fat source to your snack, such as a little peanut butter, sliced avocado, nuts, or seeds. Because fat digests slowly, this will help turn down hunger until your next meal.)

For desserts, choose those that contain:

✧ No more than 15 grams of carbohydrate

✧ 100 to 140 total calories

To calculate the amount of carbohydrate in particular foods, read the Nutrition Facts labels on packaged goods. For foods such as apples and other fruits that come without nutrition labels, consult "The *Eat Carbs, Lose Weight* Carb Chart" on page 124 for a simple way to add up your carb grams. To find out what your protein serving should look like, see "Ordering with Your Eyes—or Your Hands!" on page 130. Finally, con-

(continued on page 125)

The *Eat Carbs, Lose Weight* Substitution Rules

Consult this chart to change the *Eat Carbs* food plan into your personal food plan that includes all of your favorite foods—and none of your least-favorite foods.

For . . .	You Can Substitute . . .
Any protein food (fish, chicken, beef, pork, etc.)	The same amount of skinless chicken or turkey breast, fish, lean beef (flank steak, tenderloin, or roast beef), pork tenderloin, or lean veal or lamb chop
Any dessert (pudding, cheesecake, etc.)	¼ cup sherbet ¼ cup Tofutti ½ cup gelatin ½ cup low-fat ice cream or frozen yogurt 1 oz. fudge 1 oz. gumdrops 1 oz. peanut brittle 1 oz. pound cake 1 chocolate Pudding Pop 1 fat-free pudding cup 1 frozen fruit juice bar 1 fruit-filled cookie (0.75 oz.) 1 small brownie 1 snack-size Heath bar 1 snack-size Hershey bar 2 gingersnaps 2 graham crackers 2 oz. angel food cake 4 butterscotch pieces 5 animal crackers 7 chocolate-covered almonds 10 candy corn pieces
Any snack	Any dessert (listed above) ¼ bag microwave popcorn ¼ soft pretzel ½ banana ½ energy bar (such as a Hershey's SmartZone nutrition bar) ½ cup fruit juice ½ oz. potato chips (half of 1-oz. bag) 1 cup chopped fruit 1 small piece fruit 5 mini rice cakes

For . . .	You Can Substitute . . .
Any snack	6 to 8 oz. yogurt 15 grapes
Any fruit serving	½ mango ½ grapefruit 1 cup fresh berries 1 cup melon cubes 1 medium peach 1 small apple 1 small banana 1 small nectarine 1 small orange
Any starchy carbohydrate listed on the plan (bread, root vegetables, grains)	¼ large bagel ⅓ cup cooked barley ⅓ cup cooked couscous ⅓ cup cooked legumes ⅓ cup cooked pasta ⅓ cup cooked rice ½ English muffin ½ hamburger bun ½ cup cooked bulgur ½ cup corn ¾ cup cold, unsweetened cereal ¾-oz. bag pretzels 1 slice bread (preferably whole wheat) 3 cups air-popped popcorn 3-oz. baked potato or sweet potato
Any fat serving	2 tsp. light butter 1 tsp. cooking oil 1 tsp. regular butter 1 tsp. trans-free margarine 1 Tbsp. cream cheese 2 Tbsp. light cream cheese
Any nonstarchy vegetable (example, broccoli)*	½ cup cooked vegetable (carrots, broccoli, zucchini, cabbage, spinach, etc.) 1 cup chopped raw vegetable or salad greens

*If you need to splurge, do it here, as these vegetables are all low in calories.

The *Eat Carbs, Lose Weight* Carb Chart

On the *Eat Carbs, Lose Weight* plan, you can consume up to 45 grams of carbohydrate at breakfast, lunch, or dinner; 15 to 20 grams during your snacks; and 15 grams for dessert. Each carbohydrate serving equals 15 grams, so hold yourself to one serving for snacks and three servings for meals.

Consult the chart below to learn the serving size of various carbohydrate foods. For additional carb counts not found on this chart, consult nutrition labels on packaged foods or a carbohydrate counter, such as *The Doctor's Pocket Calorie, Fat, and Carb Counter.*

Food	Serving Size
Baked potato	½ potato
Banana	½ medium
Bread	1 slice
Chopped fruit or berries	1 cup
Corn	½ cup
Fruit juice	½ cup (4 oz.)
Grapes	12 to 15
Milk (fat-free or 1%)	1 cup (8 oz.)
Most grains (hot cereal, couscous, etc.)	½ cup cooked
Most vegetables*	½ cup cooked, 1 ½ cups uncooked
Most whole fruit (apple, orange, plum, etc.)	1 small piece, the size of your fist
Pasta	⅓ cup cooked
Rice	⅓ cup cooked
Tortilla	1 (6")
Yogurt (low-fat)	1 small container (6 to 8 oz.)

Because the following vegetables are low in calories and carbohydrates, you can splurge on these and eat more than the recommended serving size: bell peppers, broccoli, carrots, celery, cucumbers, garlic, lettuce, onions, salad greens, spinach, and tomatoes.

sult the "Adding Up Your Fat Servings" chart on page 128 for serving sizes for various types of fat and fatty foods.

THE *EAT CARBS, LOSE WEIGHT* MAINTENANCE PLAN

Do you want to become a successful maintainer? Let's look back at the 4,000 women and men on the National Weight Control Registry who have lost stunning amounts of weight and kept it off long term. When researchers at the University of Colorado and the University of Pittsburgh crunched the numbers, they learned that the average successful maintainer kept the weight off by consuming between 1,400 and 1,500 calories a day.

To lose weight on the *Eat Carbs, Lose Weight* plan, you've been eating about 1,300 daily calories. This number of calories has helped you tip that all-important weight-loss equation to the negative, ensuring that your calories in have totaled fewer than your calories out. Now, as with the successful maintainers, you want to balance that equation, so the calories you consume equal the calories you burn. To do so, you will eat about 100 to 200 calories more a day—which sounds pretty good, huh? The trick is not to overestimate the number you'll need to maintain.

So, to find the right number of calories for you, follow this three-step process.

Step 1. Record your weight. This will serve as your maintenance baseline.

Step 2. For 2 weeks, add 100 calories of the healthy foods back into your daily diet. (See "100-Calorie Foods" on page 126.) Weigh yourself and take your measurements once a week. If after 2 weeks you are still losing weight, move on to step 3. If after 2 weeks you have maintained your weight, remain at step 2. If you have gained weight, return to the *Eat Carbs, Lose Weight* weight-loss plan and continue eating roughly 1,300 calories a day.

Step 3. After 2 weeks, if you are still losing weight, add 100 more calories per day to your daily menu. Continue to weigh yourself and take your measurements once a week.

If after 2 weeks you are maintaining your weight with 200 additional calories, remain at step 3. If you are gaining weight, return to step 2.

In addition to holding themselves to roughly 1,500 daily calories, the men and women on the National Weight Control Registry also exercised 30 to 60 minutes a day—every day. Hopefully, you've been following the 12-minute Daily Dozen plan and doing your cardio walks. Now that you're in the habit of regular exercise, which is really the biggest hurdle to overcome, I strongly encourage you to increase your exercise time to 45 to 60 daily minutes. Don't let this amount of time scare you. You can easily amass this amount of exercise time by combining the following tactics.

✧ Two days a week, upgrade from the 12-minute Daily Dozen routine to a formal muscle-toning routine with weights. When you are rushed for time, traveling, or exercising somewhere where you don't have access to weights, go ahead and do the 12-minute Daily Dozen routine. That's what it's for! Most of the time, however, I'd like you to challenge your muscles more. Target your major muscle groups (chest, back, arms,

100-Calorie Foods

To add 100 calories to your daily diet, you can increase the carbohydrate portion of your breakfast, lunch, or dinner by one serving or your protein portion by two servings. For example, on Day 2 of the plan, you can increase the 4-ounce serving of chicken breast at dinner to 6 ounces or have a slice of bread along with your salad at lunch.

100-Calorie Servings	Examples
1 carbohydrate serving	⅓ cup cooked pasta
	½ potato
	1 slice whole-wheat bread
	1 small piece fruit
	8 oz. fat-free or 1% milk
2 lean protein servings	2 oz. skinless poultry, fish, or lean meat

shoulders, legs, and buns) by exercising to one of my muscle-toning DVDs, to my television show, or on your own at the gym or at home.

✧ Most days of the week, include a formal cardio session. For example, you might exercise to one of my videos, take a 30-minute power walk, or head to the gym for some time on the treadmill, stairclimber, or elliptical trainer.

✧ Try to add as many additional minutes of exercise as you can over the course of the day. For example, you might take two or more 5-minute walking breaks at work. To help clear your head, climb the stairs, do squats while you talk on the phone, or walk the dog, as I do (my Portuguese water dog, Madonna). I recommend you wear a pedometer, an inexpensive device that you hook to your waistband to record the number of steps you take in a day. Aim for 11,000 to 12,000 daily steps, which is the number the women and men in the National Weight Control Registry take on average every day. You'll be amazed how quickly those steps add up with small changes like doing leg lifts in the kitchen while cooking, taking the stairs instead of the elevator, and walking to a coworker's office instead of sending an e-mail.

In addition to monitoring your food choices and getting plenty of daily exercise, I encourage you to weigh yourself once a week for the rest of your life, as the successful maintainers in the National Weight Control Registry have done. Don't get compulsive about it—this is just to keep an eye on things. Try to stick to a range of 5 pounds—2 to 3 above your goal weight and 2 to 3 below it. This type of regular self-monitoring will help you to quickly notice whether you are gaining weight so you can modify your exercise and food consumption accordingly.

TAKING YOUR *EAT CARBS* LIFESTYLE OUTSIDE THE HOME

During the first 28 days of the *Eat Carbs, Lose Weight* plan, I strongly encourage you to prepare your own meals as often as possible and try to stick to the meal plans. As I've mentioned before, this will help you develop new habits, try new foods, and get used to a new way of eating. Beyond 28 days and during the maintenance phase of the plan, however, you'll want to eat out from time to time or go to family's or friends' homes for dinner and let other people do the cooking.

Consuming a restaurant meal every now and then will help ensure the *Eat Carbs, Lose Weight* plan conveniently fits into your lifestyle. From time to time, you may find yourself entertaining clients over dinner, for example. Every once in a while, you may realize you are just too harried to cook or that you just don't have time to shop for the ingredients you need. These are ideal reasons to eat out.

You don't, however, want to make eating out a daily habit. When you eat at home, you have the most control over what ends up on your plate and therefore over what and how much you eat. When you eat out, you are at the mercy of the chef, who, research shows, tends to dish up portions much larger than you really need to eat (not to mention drenching those bigger portions with oil or butter just before they arrive on your

Adding Up Your Fat Servings

On the *Eat Carbs, Lose Weight* plan, one serving of fat equals:
- 1 teaspoon cooking oil
- 1 teaspoon butter
- 1 teaspoon trans-free margarine
- 1 teaspoon mayonnaise
- 1 tablespoon light butter
- 1 tablespoon reduced-fat margarine or mayonnaise
- 1 tablespoon salad dressing
- 1 tablespoon cream cheese
- 2 tablespoons light cream cheese
- ⅛ avocado
- 8 large black olives
- 10 large stuffed green olives

table—just to enhance the look and flavor!). As I've mentioned before, most of us tend to eat what we see, so the typical restaurant meal can easily add up to lots of unwanted—and unneeded—calories.

By following what I call "the plate method," along with a few simple pointers, you will be able to easily stick to reasonable portions during your occasional forays to restaurants. The plate method can also give you the motivation and know-how to stick with the *Eat Carbs* plan in any situation, from holiday dinners to office parties.

Whether eating out or in, always shoot for balanced portions of carbohydrate, protein, and fat. Order meals (or dish them up) so that roughly half of your plate is covered with steamed vegetables or a salad, a quarter of your plate with another type of carbohydrate food such as a whole grain or pasta or brown rice, and the final quarter with lean protein such as chicken or salmon. You can also consume one to two servings of fat (see "Adding Up Your Fat Servings").

That said, restaurant plates vary tremendously in size. Just because the waiter brings a gargantuan plate doesn't mean you should eat all of the food that fits onto it. When the waiter brings your food, eyeball your portions and remove any excess. The first 28 days on the plan will help you do just that. With each meal, you'll actually *see* how much food you should be eating in order to lose weight and keep it off.

You can use the following guide to make sure your meal has reasonable protein, carbohydrate, vegetable, and fat portions.

Protein. This should total about 3 to 5 ounces, the size of one to two decks of cards.

Carbohydrate. This should total no more than 45 grams, which would be the same as a medium potato, a cup of pasta or other type of grain, or two slices of bread.

Vegetables. For most vegetables, you can eat more than a typical serving because they are so low in calories. If you are going to go for a larger portion, get it steamed or grilled and without extra sauces.

Fat. Your fat servings will almost always come as a sauce on top of your meat or carbohydrate portion. If you are eating your carbs and protein dry, then you can add 1 or 2 teaspoons of butter or oil (or margarine, if that's your preference) to your meal.

Consult "Ordering with Your Eyes—or Your Hands!" below or "Eyeball It" on page 136 to get a visual picture of what these portions look like.

Your restaurant meal will inevitably come with larger portions than you need. You can stay in control, however, by following these tips.

Order half portions or share. A growing number of restaurants now offer half or small portions at a reduced price. Take advantage of these, as many do resemble reasonable portions and won't tempt you to overeat. If your restaurant does not offer half portions, consider creating your own by splitting an entrée with your dining companion.

Opt for appetizers. In lieu of half portions, you can also order two or three appetizers instead of a main course. For example, you might order a grilled chicken salad along with a broth-based soup or bruschetta together with the shrimp cocktail. An added bonus: more flavors for fewer calories!

Order a custom meal. Don't be afraid to make requests. For example, see if the fish can be grilled or broiled with olive oil, rather than butter. Also, ask for any type of sauce, gravy, or dressing to be served on the side.

Make a to-go container as soon as your food arrives. If you're eating at a restaurant where the food is served in gargantuan portions, ask the waiter to bring a to-go container *with your meal.* As soon as the waiter places your plate in front of you, pare it down to reasonable portions and put the rest in the to-go container. (I've never done this, but my girlfriend who lost 40 pounds does it, and it works for her.)

Sip on a low-calorie beverage while waiting for the main course. This will help you

Ordering with Your Eyes—or Your Hands!

Use the following visuals to consume the right amount of protein, carbohydrate, or fat when eating out.

✧ 3 to 5 ounces of meat = two decks of cards, a checkbook, or the palm of a woman's hand

✧ 1 cup pasta or grain = one tennis ball or the size of a woman's fist

✧ 1 serving butter or margarine = one die or the tip of your thumb

"I Ate Carbs and Lost Weight!"

Name: Karen Niemand

Age: 43

Town: Aubonne, Switzerland

Weight Lost: 6 pounds in 4 weeks

Other Accomplishments: Lost 3 inches, dropped below 130 pounds, and feels like a new, sexier person; she's even training for a marathon

"I never lasted longer than 5 days on a diet—until now. The philosophy of low-carb diets bothered me. It drove me nuts to see a package labeled 'low carb' only to discover that the food was loaded with calories.

"Because I'm an avid runner and biker, I always ate a balanced diet, but my portions were way too big. And now that I'm older—I just turned 43—those extra calories are staying on my body. So I loved the idea of having fixed portion sizes and not just the 'eat as much as you like of one item' train of thought like some of those other diets promote.

"This diet was for me because I am a true lover of carbohydrates. I love to bake, and I'm always trying new cakes and pies. I'm quite good at it, so I have to be careful! Before *Eat Carbs, Lose Weight,* I used to crave bread and couldn't stop eating it once I started. But after only 1 to 2 days on the diet, the cravings were already gone. I didn't even want bread.

"Even though I didn't lose a whole lot of weight, I feel really good about my results. I got down below 130, which was my initial goal. The scale may not have shown weight loss right in the beginning, but my husband noticed the difference, and he was very pleased with what he saw.

"To help stay motivated, I'm going to continue to exercise. I am doing a marathon (maybe even two!) this year. I've learned that it's not so much a question of dieting for a month, because once the weight comes off, it's easy to go back to bad habits. You need to change your lifestyle and eating habits for good. I think that's what sounds so daunting for many women—the idea that it is a lifetime struggle. But I think once you integrate the changes into your life, you no longer see it as a struggle but as something natural and healthful."

Karen's advice: "Combine exercise with the eating plan. If you work out, it makes you a lot more aware of your body. If you're not sports-minded, buy a bikini and keep wearing it until you look good in it. And don't deprive yourself. If you want a croissant or a piece of chocolate, eat it and then just be more careful afterward."

find the willpower to keep your hands out of the bread or chip basket. The calories of alcoholic beverages and soft drinks can quickly add up, so opt for club soda, plain water, tomato juice, or seltzer with a spritz of fruit juice (such as cranberry and seltzer).

Send the bread back to the kitchen. Most restaurants serve some sort of free food at the beginning of the meal, such as bread or chips. Take only what you plan to eat and ask the waiter to remove the rest. It's much easier to stick to one small roll when you must physically flag down the waiter in order to get a second one.

Order one dessert for the table. It's challenging to resist a huge piece of chocolate cake when it's sitting in front of you. You might promise yourself you'll have only a few bites, but soon you may look down and see you've left only a few crumbs. On the other hand, it's much easier to savor just a few bites when you are sharing that cake with three or four other people.

If you absolutely have to stop at a fast-food restaurant, order the smallest portions possible. I'm not a big fan of fast food, as it's almost always packed with excess calories, saturated fat, and trans fat. Yet, I am a mom and know that, when traveling or pressed for time, we sometimes go there. Try to keep your consumption of fast food to a minimum. When you must stop at fast-food places, order the smallest burger or fries available and ask for water or fat-free milk instead of soda. (Wendy's now offers a salad or other healthful options with their combo meals.) If possible, choose the healthiest options from the menu, such as a salad (minus the full-fat dressing and fried bacon bits), fresh fruit, or grilled chicken sandwich.

Avoid buffet-style restaurants. As I've said before, we're only human and we tend to eat what we see. At a buffet, you will see *a lot* of food. If you must eat at a buffet for work or a family obligation, use the plate method that I mentioned earlier (filling half the plate with veggies, a quarter with carbs, and a quarter with protein). Sit down at the table so that you are facing away from the buffet. Once you finish your meal, suck on a piece of hard candy or a mint. This will keep your mouth busy and help give you the willpower to resist going up for seconds.

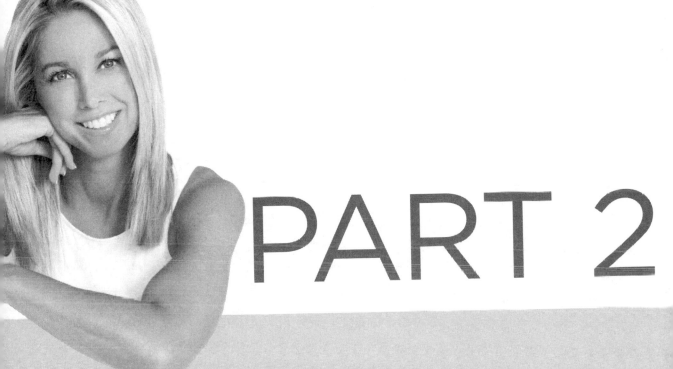

PART 2

The *Eat Carbs, Lose Weight* Diet

8

THE *EAT CARBS, LOSE WEIGHT* MENU PLAN

Learn how to turn your cravings into lost pounds and inches

Welcome to the *Eat Carbs, Lose Weight* meal plan. The next 28 days and beyond will be a true adventure. You will try many new foods and recipes. I'm confident that you will love every taste! Within the next 28 days, you will put carbs back on your plate and still lose weight. You'll enjoy your favorite sweet foods as you burn fat and see the reading on your scale go down. With the *Eat Carbs* 50–25–25 balance of carbohydrates, protein, and fat, you will feel satisfied on fewer calories, and with the meal plan's focus on high-fiber, wholesome foods, you'll boost your health and energy as you burn off the fat.

Each day, you'll find menus full of my favorite foods. Every meal contains balanced portions of carbohydrates, proteins, and fats in the optimum amounts for weight loss and blood sugar control. Each day, you'll consume the right amount of fiber and fat so you won't crave foods or feel starved. You'll also eat plenty of satisfying fiber and the optimal amount of calories to burn fat without slowing your metabolism.

I promise you, when you follow this plan, you will feel more nutritionally satisfied than you have in years. You'll see your energy levels soar, and your cravings and hunger pains will diminish. Best of all, each week when you step on the scale, you'll see your weight drop.

I'm convinced that by the end of your first 28 days on the *Eat Carbs, Lose Weight*

Eyeball It

Nutritionist Amy Campbell and I have included precise servings for each and every food you will eat during the next 28 days and beyond. If you are ever unsure of what a particular serving should look like, consult the following chart for insight.

Food Listed on the Meal Plan	What the Right Serving Looks Like
American cheese, 1 oz.	1 slice
Apple, small	Tennis ball
Bread, 1 slice	Cassette tape
Carrot, medium	7½" long
Cheddar cheese, 1 oz.	Your thumb (tip to base)
Chicken breast, 2 oz. sliced	Slightly smaller than your palm
Chicken, 4 oz.	Your palm
Ham, 3 oz. sliced	Your palm
Kiwifruit, large	Your fist
Milk, orange juice, tomato juice; 4 oz.	One cupped handful
Milk, orange juice, tomato juice; 8 oz.	Two cupped handfuls
Orange, small	Baseball
Peach, medium	Your fist
Pear, medium	Your fist
Potato, baked medium	Computer mouse
String cheese, 1 oz.	Three dice
Sweet potato, baked medium	Computer mouse
Tangerine, medium	Your fist
Turkey breast, 3 oz. sliced	Your palm

plan, you'll feel as enthusiastic as I do about this way of eating for weight loss. Don't forget to write down your initial measurements and weight. Step on the scale first thing in the morning and write down the number that you see pop up. Then, with a flexible tape measure, take your waist measurement. For fun and motivation, you can also take your hip, thigh, and bust measurements. (See chapter 7 for advice on taking your measurements and picking a goal weight.) Once you start the plan, I recommend you record your weight and measurements once a week, ideally at the same time of day. You might write down and post your ongoing results at a motivational location that you will see often.

For optimum success, follow these pointers.

✧ Measure out your ingredients and snacks with measuring cups and spoons. As you dish up each meal or snack, make a mental note of what each meal looks like on your plate. This will help you to more easily maintain your success later on. Portions are important.

✧ Switch to a smaller dinner plate. This will visually trick your brain into thinking you are eating more food. In this way, you'll mentally feel more satisfied after each meal.

✧ When you dish up your meals, do so in the kitchen and then carry your plate to the table. If possible, put away the leftovers before you start eating. This will help ensure you don't go back for seconds.

✧ When you store leftovers in your refrigerator or freezer, dish them into small containers in the correct portions. In this way, you will create your own fresh or frozen meals in the right portions for weight loss.

✧ Portion out your snacks the night before you need them. For example, if the next day's snack calls for 20 peanuts, put 20 peanuts in a bag. This will help you avoid mindless grazing that can add up to hundreds of excess calories.

✧ To get a mental picture of the serving size for beverages, use the same drinking glass every day. Measure out both a 4-ounce serving and an 8-ounce serving of liquid. Dump one at a time into the glass and use a permanent marker to mark a

4-ounce line and an 8-ounce line on the outside of the glass. Once you've marked your glass, you'll always know how much to pour.

✧ At the beginning of each week, look over the meal plan for the week to come and make your shopping list.

✧ If you find yourself needing to swap one day for another, that's fine. Sometimes, based on what's in the refrigerator or what's going on in our lives, it's easier to repeat or omit a day here or there. Just don't follow the same day more than two times during the plan—the nutritional variety is one way the plan helps you lose weight and optimize your health, and trying all the recipes may introduce you to a food you never knew you could love!

Are you excited to embark on this revolutionary way of eating? I sure hope you are! I'm convinced that you will love the *Eat Carbs* plan as much as I do. Think of your first day on the plan as a fresh start to the rest of your life. You'll lose weight, look fantastic, and feel wonderful. Better health. Trimmer thighs. More energy. Radiant skin. What are you waiting for? Turn the page and get started on your journey to a new you!

DAY 1

Meal/Snack	Calories	Carbs (g)	Protein (g)	Fat (g)	Fiber (g)	Sodium (mg)
BREAKFAST						
1 Breakfast Burrito (page 170)	290	32	13	12	6	480
½ medium grapefruit	53	13	1	0	2	0
SNACK						
1 medium pear	62	16	0	0	3	0
LUNCH						
1¼ cups Country Garden Gazpacho with Garlic Croutons (page 188)	130	21	4	4.5	4	450
¼ cup Hummus with Roasted Red Peppers (page 189)	87	14	4	3	3	130
1 oz. low-fat Cheddar cheese	49	0	7	2	0	174
4 (4") carrot sticks	15	3	0	0	1	0
2 celery ribs	20	5	1	0	2	11
SNACK						
½ cup cook-and-serve pudding	150	22	1	0	1	110
DINNER						
3 oz. broiled lean tenderloin steak	197	0	24	11	0	54
2 servings Baked Spinach-Stuffed Potatoes (page 211)	200	32	10	2	2	320
1 cup steamed summer squash	36	8	2	0	3	2
2 tsp. light whipped butter	24	0	0	2	0	3
Total:	**1,313**	**166**	**67**	**36.5**	**27**	**1,734**
		51%	20%	25%*		

You may notice that the percentages for carbs, protein, and fat do not always add up to 100. That's because of mathematical rounding done during nutrient calculations. Not to worry—the entire plan features balanced nutrition by day and by week.

DAY 2

Meal/Snack	Calories	Carbs (g)	Protein (g)	Fat (g)	Fiber (g)	Sodium (mg)
BREAKFAST						
1 Coffee-Chocolate Waffle (page 171)	235	29	10	10	5	400
1 Tbsp. lower-calorie maple syrup	15	4	0	0	0	26
1 cup blueberries	70	16	0	0	4	10
SNACK						
6 oz. light yogurt	100	17	5	0	0	85
LUNCH						
1 serving Greek-Style Vegetable Salad (page 190)	338	34	12	18	8	1,040
SNACK						
1 small apple	63	16	0	0	3	0
DINNER						
⅔ cup cooked brown rice	144	30	3	1	2	7
2 tsp. light whipped butter	24	0	0	2	0	3
¾ cup Sautéed Zucchini with Garlic and Parsley (page 212)	50	4	1	4	1	160
4 (4") carrot sticks	15	3	0	0	0	0
4 oz. baked skinless chicken breast	187	0	35	4	0	84
1 frozen fruit juice bar	45	11	0	0	0	0
Total:	**1,286**	**164**	**66**	**39**	**23**	**1,815**
		51%	21%	27%		

DAY 3

Meal/Snack	Calories	Carbs (g)	Protein (g)	Fat (g)	Fiber (g)	Sodium (mg)
BREAKFAST 1½ cups Fruity Ginger Smoothie (page 172)	191	42	4	3	4	42
SNACK 1 small apple	63	16	0	0	3	0
7 walnut halves	93	2	2	9	1	0
LUNCH 2 slices multigrain bread	120	24	6	1	4	240
4 oz. water-packed tuna, rinsed	120	0	28	4	0	60
2 Tbsp. light mayonnaise	100	2	0	10	0	230
½ small tomato, sliced; green leaf lettuce	13	3	0.5	0	1	6
8 oz. fat-free milk	86	12	8	0	0	127
SNACK 2 popcorn cakes	77	16	2	1	1	58
1 Tbsp. peanut butter	95	3.5	4	8	1	75
DINNER 1 serving Brown Rice and Tangy Beans (page 213)	208	40	7	5	8	600
1 cup steamed broccoli	44	8	5	1	5	41
1 small tomato, sliced	20	5	0	0	1	0
2 tsp. olive oil	80	0	0	9	0	0
Total:	**1,310**	**173.5**	**66.5**	**51**	**29**	**1,479**
		53%	20%	35%		

DAY 4

Meal/Snack	Calories	Carbs (g)	Protein (g)	Fat (g)	Fiber (g)	Sodium (mg)
BREAKFAST						
½ cup cooked oatmeal	66	13	2	1	1	104
8 oz. fat-free milk	86	12	8	0	0	127
2 Tbsp. raisins	65	16	0.5	0	1	0
2 Tbsp. chopped walnuts	95	2	4	9	1	5
SNACK						
1 cup frozen papaya chunks	55	14	1	0	3	4
LUNCH						
1 Turkey-Veggie Pita (page 191)	391	42	33	17	7	461
4 oz. reduced-sodium tomato juice	17	4	1	0	1	6
SNACK						
6 oz. light yogurt	100	17	5	0	0	85
DINNER						
1 serving Lime-Grilled Chicken with Cuban Salsa (page 214)	290	22	37	5	5	620
⅓ cup cooked brown rice	72	15	2	1	1	3
½ cup sliced mushrooms	10	2	0	0	0	0
2 Pecan Crisps (page 252)	126	12	2	8	12	0
Total:	**1,373**	**171**	**95.5**	**41**	**32**	**1,415**
		50%	28%	27%		

DAY 5

Meal/Snack	Calories	Carbs (g)	Protein (g)	Fat (g)	Fiber (g)	Sodium (mg)
BREAKFAST						
1 cup puffed Kashi cereal	70	19	3	1	2	0
8 oz. fat-free milk	86	12	8	0	0	127
½ cup fresh berries	35	8	0	0	2	5
2 Tbsp. sunflower seeds	103	3	4	9	2	1
SNACK						
5 dried apple rings	78	21	0	0	3	28
LUNCH						
1 Smoked Turkey, Arugula, and Cranberry Wrap (page 192)	331	39	26	9	4	1,120
1 cup cherry tomatoes	20	5	0	0	1	0
1 cup raw broccoli florets	20	4	2	0	0	0
SNACK						
3 cups air-popped popcorn	92	19	3	1	4	1
2 Tbsp. Parmesan cheese, plus optional chili powder	46	0	4	3	0	186
DINNER						
3 oz. broiled pork tenderloin	120	0	17	5	0	40
1 serving Roasted Asparagus and Mixed Vegetables (page 215)	199	31	9	5	8	420
½ baked medium sweet potato	59	14	1	0	2	6
1 Tbsp. light whipped butter	35	0	0	3	0	4.5
Total:	**1,294**	**175**	**77**	**36**	**28**	**1,938.5**
		54%	24%	25%		

DAY 6

Meal/Snack	Calories	Carbs (g)	Protein (g)	Fat (g)	Fiber (g)	Sodium (mg)
BREAKFAST						
1 whole-wheat English muffin	134	27	6	1	4	420
1 Tbsp. light whipped butter	35	0	0	3	0	4.5
2 tsp. all-fruit spread	4	2	0	0	0	4
8 oz. fat-free milk	86	12	8	0	0	127
SNACK						
1 medium peach	42	11	1	0	2	0
LUNCH						
½ cup Slim Sloppy Joes (page 193)	150	21	12	3.5	3	470
1 whole-wheat hamburger bun	117	22	3.5	2	3	256
1 cup cucumber and carrot sticks	15	3	0	0	0	0
1 small tomato, sliced	20	5	0	0	1	0
15 grapes	62	15	0	0	1	2
SNACK						
22 almonds	169	5	6	15	3	96
1 medium tangerine	37	9	0.5	0	2	1
DINNER						
1 serving Chicken-Cashew Toss on Greens (page 216)	286	18	24	11	4	670
1 small whole-wheat dinner roll	75	14	2	1	2	135
2 tsp. light butter	24	0	0	2	0	3
1 frozen fruit juice bar	45	11	0	0	0	0
Total:	**1,301**	**175**	**63**	**38.5**	**25**	**2,188.5**
		54%	**19%**	**27%**		

DAY 7

Meal/Snack	Calories	Carbs (g)	Protein (g)	Fat (g)	Fiber (g)	Sodium (mg)
BREAKFAST 2 Tbsp. Smoked Salmon Spread with 2 slices pumpernickel bread (page 173)	134	20	5	4	3	311
½ medium grapefruit	53	13	1	0	2	0
SNACK 6 oz. light yogurt	100	17	5	0	0	85
LUNCH 2 cups Hearty Herbed Chicken Soup (page 194)	323	21	48	5	5	1,490
3 Stoned Wheat Thins crackers	90	15	3	2	2	210
4 (4") carrot sticks	15	3	0	0	1	0
1 cup cucumber sticks	10	2	0	0	0	0
SNACK 2 plums	73	17	1	1	2	0
DINNER 4 oz. broiled/grilled salmon	206	0	29	9	0	63
1 serving Maple-Mashed Sweet Potatoes (page 217)	130	31	2	0	4	50
1 cup brussels sprouts	61	14	4	1	4	33
1 tsp. olive oil	40	0	0	5	0	0
Total:	**1,235**	**153**	**98**	**27**	**23**	**2,242**
		50%	32%	20%		

DAY 8

Meal/Snack	Calories	Carbs (g)	Protein (g)	Fat (g)	Fiber (g)	Sodium (mg)
BREAKFAST						
1 serving Whole-Wheat French Toast with Fresh Strawberries (page 174)	270	38	11	10	4	300
SNACK						
6 dried apricots	50	13	1	0	2	2
LUNCH						
1 Avocado Quesadilla (page 195)	270	29	12	13	5	783
1 cup raw broccoli florets	20	4	2	0	0	0
1 frozen fruit juice bar	45	11	0	0	0	0
SNACK						
6 oz. light yogurt	100	17	5	0	0	85
2 tsp. ground flaxseed	40	2	2	2	2	2
DINNER						
4 oz. baked skinless chicken breast	187	0	35	4	0	84
1 serving Buttermilk Mashed Spuds with Garlic and Leeks (page 218)	165	19	7	8	5	270
1 serving Sautéed Red Peppers with Balsamic Vinegar and Almonds (page 219)	90	8	2	6	2	150
1 baked apple with cinnamon and	63	16	0	0	3	0
1 tsp. brown sugar	17	4	0	0	0	2
Total:	**1,317**	**161**	**77**	**43**	**23**	**1,678**
		49%	**23%**	**29%**		

DAY 9

Meal/Snack	Calories	Carbs (g)	Protein (g)	Fat (g)	Fiber (g)	Sodium (mg)
BREAKFAST						
1 serving Western Scramble (page 175)	170	14	13	7	2	400
1 slice whole-wheat toast	69	13	3	1	2	148
2 tsp. light whipped butter	24	0	0	2	0	3
4 oz. calcium-fortified orange juice	55	13	1	0	0	0
SNACK						
½ cup pineapple chunks	70	17	0	0	1	10
LUNCH						
1 cup tomato-vegetable soup	100	19	3	1.5	2	660
2 RyKrisp crackers	73	16	2	0	3	53
½ cup shredded part-skim mozzarella	135	0	12	9	0	330
1 cup celery sticks	20	5	1	0	2	108
1 Tbsp. peanut butter	95	3.5	4	8	1	75
SNACK						
¼ cup unsweetened applesauce	29	8	0	0	0	0
2 Tbsp. low-fat granola	53	11	1	1	1	34
DINNER						
1 serving Tropical Salad with Baby Greens (page 220)	129	12	2	9	4	220
1 serving Steak and Bell Pepper Fajitas (page 221)	308	32	29	9	4	700
1 cup cherry tomatoes	20	5	0	0	1	0
Total:	**1,350**	**168.5**	**71**	**47.5**	**23**	**2,741**
		50%	21%	32%		

DAY 10

Meal/Snack	Calories	Carbs (g)	Protein (g)	Fat (g)	Fiber (g)	Sodium (mg)
BREAKFAST						
1 Double-A Applesauce Muffin (page 176)	100	19	2	2	3	115
2 Tbsp. almond butter	220	3	8	19	0	10
4 oz. calcium-fortified orange juice	55	13	1	0	0	0
SNACK						
4 oz. light yogurt	67	11	3	0	0	57
1 Tbsp. raisins	33	8	0	0	1	3
LUNCH						
1 serving Shrimp and Avocados with Chiles and Lime (page 196)	296	15	27	16	7	570
½ cup cut green and red peppers	12	3	0	0	0	0
1 small whole-wheat roll	75	14	2	1	2	135
½ cup cantaloupe chunks	28	7	0.5	0	1	7
SNACK						
11 small organic oat bran pretzels	73	15	2	0	1	196
DINNER						
1 serving Baked Chicken Thighs with Chickpeas and Tomatoes (page 222)	240	25	18	7	5	590
2 cups salad, with red leaf lettuce	20	4	1	0	1	13
1 Tbsp. light Italian dressing	7	1	0	0.5	0	212
1 serving Pineapple Mexicali (page 253)	74	19	1	0	3	2
Total:	1,300	157	65.5	45.5	24	1,910
		48%	20%	32%		

DAY 11

Meal/Snack	Calories	Carbs (g)	Protein (g)	Fat (g)	Fiber (g)	Sodium (mg)
BREAKFAST 1½ cups Fruity Ginger Smoothie (page 172)	191	42	4	3	4	42
SNACK 1 medium tangerine	37	9	0.5	0	2	1
20 peanuts, no salt added	117	4	5	10	2	1
LUNCH 1 Pepperoni Pita Pizza (page 197)	241	27	13	9	4	704
4 (4") carrot sticks	15	3	0	0	1	0
4 (4") zucchini sticks	13	3	0	0	1	0
½ cup cook-and-serve pudding	150	22	1	0	1	110
SNACK 2 popcorn cakes	77	16	2	1	1	58
DINNER 1 serving Pork Tenderloin and Vegetable Stir-Fry (page 223)	267	16	26	10	3	580
1 serving Veggie Rice with Egg (page 224)	228	32	6	9	4	530
Total:	1,336	174	57.5	42	23	2,026
		52%	17%	28%		

DAY 12

Meal/Snack	Calories	Carbs (g)	Protein (g)	Fat (g)	Fiber (g)	Sodium (mg)
BREAKFAST						
1 cup Fruity Oatmeal (page 177)	200	37	8	3.5	5	65
¼ cup fat-free milk	21	3	2	0	0	32
1 tsp. honey	20	5	0	0	0	0
1 tsp. ground flaxseed	20	1	1	1	1	1
1 slice Canadian bacon	50	0	8	1	0	620
SNACK						
10 sweet cherries	49	11	1	1	2	0
LUNCH						
1 whole-wheat hamburger roll	117	22	3.5	2	3	256
1 veggie burger	94	7	16	0	3	369
1 slice low-fat American cheese	40	2	5	1	0	200
Green leaf lettuce; 2 tomato slices	11	2.5	0	0	1	5
1 Tbsp. mayonnaise	100	0	0	11	0	80
½ cup cantaloupe chunks	28	7	0.5	0	1	7
SNACK						
Gorp made with 2 tsp. raisins, 2 tsp. chocolate chips, 2 tsp. sunflower seeds, and 10 peanuts	166	14	4	11	4	12
DINNER						
1 serving Super "Bowlful" Chili (page 225)	227	29	17	5	10	680
½ cup steamed spinach	21	2	0	0	1	0
1 serving Glazed Pear Snack Cake (page 254)	140	24	3	4.5	2	190
Total:	**1,304**	**166.5**	**69**	**41**	**33**	**2,517**
		51%	21%	28%		

DAY 13

Meal/Snack	Calories	Carbs (g)	Protein (g)	Fat (g)	Fiber (g)	Sodium (mg)
BREAKFAST						
1 BLT Sandwich (page 178)	366	48	21	13	6	965
4 oz. calcium-fortified orange juice	55	13	1	0	0	0
SNACK						
6 oz. light yogurt	100	17	5	0	0	85
LUNCH						
Tortilla Crisps with Mashed Beans and Avocado (page 198)	247	34	12	7	9	790
1 small tomato, sliced	20	5	0	0	1	0
1 cup watermelon cubes	45	11	1	1	1	3
SNACK						
1 small apple	63	16	0	0	3	0
DINNER						
1 serving Chicken Tenders and Broccoli Stir-Fry (page 226)	351	25	30	15	7	710
½ cup raw green pepper slices	12	3	0	0	1	0
1 serving Fruit Kebabs with Honey-Mint Sauce (page 255)	100	23	2	0	1	30
Total:	1,359	195	72	36	29	2,583
		57%	21%	24%		

DAY 14

Meal/Snack	Calories	Carbs (g)	Protein (g)	Fat (g)	Fiber (g)	Sodium (mg)
BREAKFAST						
1 Breakfast Parfait (page 179)	230	37	10	7	10	134
SNACK						
1 medium tangerine	37	9	0.5	0	2	1
LUNCH						
1 Chutney Chicken Wrap (page 199)	269	30	23	6	2	471
¼ cup chopped cucumber	2	0	0	0	0	0
¼ cup sliced radishes	5	1	0	0	0	0
8 oz. fat-free milk	86	12	8	0	0	127
SNACK						
1 medium kiwifruit	46	11	1	0	3	4
1 oz. part-skim string cheese	90	2	7	6	0	200
DINNER						
1 serving Sesame Noodles with Salmon (page 227)	439	40	28	18	6	500
½ cup steamed broccoli	12	3	0	0	2	0
1 serving Peach Melba (page 256)	90	16	1	3	2	0
Total:	**1,306**	**161**	**80**	**42**	**29**	**1,457**
		49%	25%	29%		

DAY 15

Meal/Snack	Calories	Carbs (g)	Protein (g)	Fat (g)	Fiber (g)	Sodium (mg)
BREAKFAST						
3 Almond Cloud Pancakes with Peaches (page 180)	210	21	13	8	1	280
8 oz. fat-free milk	86	12	8	0	0	127
SNACK						
1 large kiwifruit	56	14	1	0	3	5
LUNCH						
2 slices multigrain bread	120	24	6	1	4	240
3 oz. sliced turkey breast	135	3	24	6	0	60
Green leaf lettuce; ½ small tomato, sliced	13	3	0.5	0	1	6
4 (4") carrot sticks	15	3	0	0	1	0
1 Tbsp. light mayonnaise	50	1	0	5	0	115
1 cup sliced strawberries	50	12	1	1	4	2
SNACK						
2 multigrain rice cakes	70	14	1.5	1	0.5	45
1 Tbsp. peanut butter	95	3.5	4	8	1	75
DINNER						
2 cups Red Wine and Beef Soup (page 229)	230	15	26	7	3	670
2 multigrain crispbread crackers	90	16	4	0	4	170
2 cups salad with baby spinach	20	4	1	0	1	13
2 Tbsp. light Italian dressing	14	2	0	1	0	424
1 cup fresh fruit salad	56	13	1	0	1	14
Total:	1,310	160.5	91	38	24.5	2,246
		49%	28%	26%		

DAY 16

Meal/Snack	Calories	Carbs (g)	Protein (g)	Fat (g)	Fiber (g)	Sodium (mg)
BREAKFAST						
1 serving Canadian Bacon and Vegetable Hash (page 181)	100	16	4	3	3	320
1 poached egg	75	0	6	5	0	140
1 slice whole-grain toast	70	13	5	0.5	5	70
2 tsp. light whipped butter	24	0	0	2	0	3
½ medium grapefruit	53	13	1	0	2	0
SNACK						
10 sweet cherries	49	11	1	1	2	0
LUNCH						
1 serving Baked Potato and Broccoli (page 200)	229	33	21	6	10	504
1 frozen fruit juice bar	45	11	0	0	0	0
SNACK						
4 oz. light yogurt	67	11	3	0	0	57
1 Tbsp. low-fat granola	27	6	1	0	0	17
DINNER						
1 serving Teriyaki Salmon with Scallion-Cucumber Relish (page 231)	220	3	29	9	0	450
1 serving Mushrooms Stuffed with Rice and Greens (page 232)	260	30	10	12	7	250
4 cherry tomatoes	16	2	0	0	1	0
1 cup sliced strawberries	50	12	1	1	4	2
1 Tbsp. light whipped topping	10	1	0	0.5	0	0
Total:	**1,295**	**162**	**82**	**40**	**34**	**1,813**
		50%	25%	28%		

DAY 17

Meal/Snack	Calories	Carbs (g)	Protein (g)	Fat (g)	Fiber (g)	Sodium (mg)
BREAKFAST						
1 whole-wheat English muffin	134	27	6	1	4	420
½ cup 1% cottage cheese	81	3	14	1	0	459
¼ small cantaloupe	48	12	1	0	1	12
1 Tbsp. light whipped butter	35	0	0	3	0	4.5
SNACK						
15 grapes	62	15	0	0	1	2
LUNCH						
1½ cups Mediterranean Tuna Salad (page 201)	330	26	26	14	5	790
½ medium oat-bran pita bread	65	15	3	0	2	150
1 cup celery sticks	20	5	1	0	2	180
SNACK						
3 cups air-popped popcorn	92	19	3	1	4	1
2 Tbsp. Parmesan cheese	46	0	4	3	0	186
DINNER						
4 oz. broiled pork tenderloin	160	0	23	7	0	53
1 serving Sautéed Green Beans with Cherry Tomatoes and Onion (page 233)	90	16	3	2.5	4	160
1 Mixed-Berry Cobbler (page 257)	83	16	1	2	3	1
2 Tbsp. light whipped topping	20	2	0	1	0	0
Total:	**1,266**	**156**	**85**	**35.5**	**26**	**2,418.5**
		49%	27%	25%		

DAY 18

Meal/Snack	Calories	Carbs (g)	Protein (g)	Fat (g)	Fiber (g)	Sodium (mg)
BREAKFAST						
1 cup puffed Kashi cereal	70	19	3	1	2	0
8 oz. fat-free milk	86	12	8	0	0	127
½ banana	46	12	0.5	0	1	5
2 Tbsp. walnuts	95	2	4	9	1	0
SNACK						
1 cup honeydew melon chunks	60	16	1	0	1	17
LUNCH						
1 Tuna Melt (page 202)	401	31	42	11	5	1,351
4 (4") carrot sticks	15	3	0	0	1	0
1 plum	36	9	1	0	1	0
SNACK						
1 Fat-Free Fudgsicle	60	12	2	0	0	40
DINNER						
1 serving Broiled Beef Slices with Bangkok Salad (page 234)	223	11	22	11	3	735
1 small whole-wheat dinner roll	75	14	2	1	2	135
¾ cup Tropical Ambrosia (page 258)	89	20	2	1	3	13
Total:	**1,256**	**161**	**87.5**	**34**	**20**	**2,423**
		51%	**28%**	**24%**		

DAY 19

Meal/Snack	Calories	Carbs (g)	Protein (g)	Fat (g)	Fiber (g)	Sodium (mg)
BREAKFAST						
½ cup cooked oatmeal	66	13	2	1	1	104
2 Tbsp. raisins	65	16	0.5	0	1	5
2 Tbsp. walnuts	95	2	4	9	1	0
8 oz. fat-free milk	86	12	8	0	0	127
SNACK						
15 grapes	62	15	0	0	1	2
1 oz. part-skim string cheese	90	2	7	6	0	200
LUNCH						
1 serving Bacon and Clam Chowder (page 203)	169	20	14	5	4	770
1 slice whole-wheat toast	69	13	3	1	2	148
2 tsp. light butter	24	0	0	2	0	3
1 medium carrot, cut into sticks	26	6	1	0	2	21
½ cucumber, cut into spears	10	2	0	0	0	0
SNACK						
2 multigrain rice cakes	70	14	1.5	1	0.5	45
1 Tbsp. peanut butter	95	3.5	4	8	1	75
DINNER						
1 serving Chile and Corn Strata (page 235)	200	20	16	8	2	120
2 cups salad with baby spinach	20	4	1	0	1	13
2 Tbsp. Italian dressing	92	3	0	9	0	560
½ cup mushrooms	10	2	0	0	0	0
1 serving Sautéed Bananas with Spiced Yogurt Topping (page 259)	120	24	2	3	2	15
Total:	**1,369**	**171.5**	**64**	**53**	**18.5**	**2,208**
		50%	19%	35%		

DAY 20

Meal/Snack	Calories	Carbs (g)	Protein (g)	Fat (g)	Fiber (g)	Sodium (mg)
BREAKFAST						
1 Fruit-Soy Smoothie (page 182)	236	39	12	4	5	111
SNACK						
10 small Ak-Mak crackers	70	14	1	0	4	0
1 Tbsp. peanut butter	95	3.5	4	8	1	75
LUNCH						
1 serving Southwestern Corn and Sweet Potato Soup (page 204)	161	30	4	5	5	680
1 cup salad with romaine lettuce	10	2	1	0	1	7
½ cup sliced radishes	10	2	0	0	0	0
2 Tbsp. light Italian dressing	14	2	0	1	0	424
1 cup cantaloupe cubes	56	14	2	0	2	14
SNACK						
1 medium kiwifruit	46	11	1	0	3	4
20 peanuts	117	4	5	10	2	1
DINNER						
1 serving Curried Chicken with Almonds and Currants (page 236)	305	22	31	9	6	510
1 cup steamed broccoli	44	8	5	1	5	41
1 serving Exotic Mushrooms with Madeira (page 237)	115	12	6	3	3	310
Total:	**1,279**	**163.5**	**72**	**41**	**37**	**2,177**
		51%	23%	29%		

DAY 21

Meal/Snack	Calories	Carbs (g)	Protein (g)	Fat (g)	Fiber (g)	Sodium (mg)
BREAKFAST						
¾ cup bran flakes	96	24	3	1	5	220
4 oz. fat-free milk	43	6	4	0	0	64
½ small banana, sliced	46	12	0.5	0	1	5
1 hard-boiled egg	78	0	6	5	0	62
SNACK						
1 large kiwifruit	56	14	1	0	3	5
30 dry-roasted peanuts	190	7	8	16	2	150
LUNCH						
1 Roasted Veggie Sandwich (page 205)	310	45	11	12	9	680
1 cup cucumber and carrot sticks	15	3	0	0	0	0
SNACK						
15 frozen green grapes	62	15	0	0	1	2
1 oz. part-skim string cheese	90	2	7	6	0	200
DINNER						
4 oz. broiled haddock	121	0	26	2	0	383
1 serving Herb-Roasted Idaho Potato Fries (page 238)	110	21	2	2.5	2	150
1 cup steamed green beans	40	8	2	0	2	10
1 serving Broiled Plum Tomatoes Parmesan (page 239)	50	4	2	3.5	1	190
Total:	**1,307**	**161**	**72.5**	**48**	**26**	**2,121**
		49%	22%	33%		

DAY 22

Meal/Snack	Calories	Carbs (g)	Protein (g)	Fat (g)	Fiber (g)	Sodium (mg)
BREAKFAST						
1 Quick Apple-Pecan Waffle (page 183)	198	30	5	6	3	259
SNACK						
1 small orange	45	11	1	0	2	0
LUNCH						
1 cup Carrot and Pea Salad (page 206)	150	27	5	3	6	125
½ cup 1% cottage cheese	81	3	14	1	0	459
3 oz. extra-lean ham	74	0	11	3	0	810
2 multigrain crispbreads	90	16	4	0	4	170
1 cup cucumber sticks	10	2	0	0	0	0
SNACK						
3 graham crackers	89	16	1.5	2	1	127
1 Tbsp. peanut butter	95	3.5	4	8	1	75
DINNER						
1 serving Turkey and Spinach Baked Peppers (page 240)	186	15	11	9	3	390
2 cups salad with romaine lettuce	20	4	1	0	1	13
½ cup artichoke hearts	38	8	3	0	4	45
2 Tbsp. light Italian dressing	14	2	0	1	0	424
1 serving Orange-Scented Cornmeal Cake with Fresh Berries (page 260)	189	30	4	7	3	200
Total:	**1,279**	**167.5**	**64.5**	**40**	**28**	**3,097**
		52%	20%	28%		

DAY 23

Meal/Snack	Calories	Carbs (g)	Protein (g)	Fat (g)	Fiber (g)	Sodium (mg)
BREAKFAST						
2 servings French Toast Soufflé with Maple Cream Topping (page 184)	300	34	18	10	2	520
1 small orange, separated into segments	45	11	1	0	2	0
SNACK						
1 cup honeydew melon chunks	60	16	1	0	1	17
LUNCH						
1 medium oat-bran pita bread	130	30	6	1	3	300
1 veggie burger	94	7	16	0	3	369
1 slice low-fat American cheese	40	2	5	1	0	200
2 tomato slices; green leaf lettuce	11	2.5	0	0	1	5
1 Tbsp. mayonnaise	100	0	0	11	0	80
SNACK						
1 cup raw broccoli florets	20	4	2	0	0	0
2 Tbsp. fat-free Ranch dressing	50	11	0	0	1	350
DINNER						
1 serving Sesame Crusted Catfish with Creamy Salsa (page 241)	190	7	27	6	2	530
1 serving Chili Potato Wedges (page 242)	109	12	5	5	6	610
4 (4") zucchini/summer squash sticks	13	3	0	0	1	0
1 serving Apple Crumble with Oat Crust (page 262)	170	32	2	4.5	3	5
1 Tbsp. light whipped topping	10	1	0	0.5	0	0
Total:	1,342	172.5	83	39	25	2,986
		51%	25%	26%		

DAY 24

Meal/Snack	Calories	Carbs (g)	Protein (g)	Fat (g)	Fiber (g)	Sodium (mg)
BREAKFAST						
½ cup Kashi cereal	95	18	4	1.5	4	45
8 oz. fat-free milk	86	12	8	0	0	127
½ small banana, sliced	46	12	0.5	0	1	5
SNACK						
1 large kiwifruit	56	14	1	0	3	5
LUNCH						
2 slices multigrain bread	120	24	6	1	4	240
3 oz. extra-lean ham	74	0	11	3	0	810
1 oz. Swiss cheese	108	0	8	9	0	39
2 tomato slices; green leaf lettuce	11	2.5	0	0	1	5
2 tsp. mustard	8	2	0	0	0	4
1 cup papaya cubes	55	14	1	0	3	4
SNACK						
1 slice Banana Nut Bread (page 263)	140	25	3	4	2	190
2 tsp. light whipped butter	24	0	0	2	0	3
DINNER						
1 serving Vegetable Frittata (page 243)	150	9	11	8	2	320
⅛ avocado	77	3	1	8	2	5
½ cup raw mushrooms	10	2	0	0	0	0
1 slice Italian bread	77	14	2	1	1	166
2 tsp. light butter	34	0	0	2	0	0
1 serving Pears Baked in Rum Cream Sauce (page 264)	110	19	4	3	2	75
Total:	**1,281**	**170.5**	**60.5**	**42.5**	**25**	**2,043**
		53%	19%	30%		

DAY 25

Meal/Snack	Calories	Carbs (g)	Protein (g)	Fat (g)	Fiber (g)	Sodium (mg)
BREAKFAST 1 Sausage and Cheese Scone (page 185)	156	16	7	7	2	388
4 oz. calcium-fortified orange juice	55	13	1	0	0	0
SNACK 1 cup papaya cubes	55	14	1	0	3	4
LUNCH 1 serving Romaine Salad with Pita Crisps and Sesame (page 207)	154	18	5	8	4	220
2 oz. deli-sliced chicken breast	94	0	18	2	0	42
½ cup yellow pepper slices	12	3	0	0	1	0
6 oz. light yogurt	100	17	5	0	0	85
¼ cup sliced strawberries	12	3	0	0	1	0
SNACK 2 Tbsp. Mexicali-Spiced Almonds (page 205)	110	4	4	9	2	10
DINNER 1 serving Spaghetti with Veggies and Tofu (page 244)	320	44	16	11	7	560
2 cups salad with red leaf lettuce	20	4	1	0	1	13
2 Tbsp. Dijon vinaigrette dressing	120	2	0	12	0	342
Total:	1,208	138	58	49	21	1,664
		46%	19%	37%		

DAY 26

Meal/Snack	Calories	Carbs (g)	Protein (g)	Fat (g)	Fiber (g)	Sodium (mg)
BREAKFAST						
1 Fruit-Soy Smoothie (page 182)	236	39	12	4	5	111
SNACK						
15 grapes	62	15	0	0	1	2
1 hard-boiled egg	78	0	6	5	0	62
LUNCH						
Veggie Soft Taco (page 208)	273	41	12	8	11	809
SNACK						
½ cup pineapple chunks	70	17	0	0	1	10
10 almonds	69	2	3	6	1	0
DINNER						
1 serving Braised Chicken Drumsticks (page 245)	276	18	28	9	4	670
1 serving Romaine and Apple Salad with Blue Cheese (page 246)	127	13	2	8	3	802
½ cup raw mushrooms	10	2	0	0	0	0
1 serving Gingered Pumpkin Pudding (page 266)	90	11	4	3.5	2	200
Total:	**1,291**	**158**	**67**	**43.5**	**27.5**	**2,666**
		49%	**21%**	**30%**		

DAY 27

Meal/Snack	Calories	Carbs (g)	Protein (g)	Fat (g)	Fiber (g)	Sodium (mg)
BREAKFAST						
2 slices whole-wheat toast	138	26	5	2	4	295
½ cup scrambled egg whites (or egg substitute)	60	2	10	2	0	180
1 Tbsp. light ketchup	8	2	0	0	0	115
½ medium grapefruit	53	13	1	0	2	0
SNACK						
4 oz. light yogurt	67	11	3	0	0	57
1 Tbsp. raisins	33	8	0	0	1	5
LUNCH						
2 slices Broccoli and Sun-Dried Tomato Quick Bread (page 209)	240	26	10	12	4	500
½ cup 1% cottage cheese	81	3	14	1	0	459
4 (4") zucchini sticks	13	3	0	0	1	0
½ cup pineapple chunks	70	17	0	0	1	10
SNACK						
3 gingersnaps	90	14	1	3	0	72
DINNER						
1 serving Turkey Meatloaf (page 247)	290	15	28	13	2	565
1 serving Balsamic-Glazed Fall Vegetables (page 248)	173	31	4	5	6	580
2 cups salad, with baby spinach	20	4	1	0	1	13
1 tsp. balsamic vinegar	3	1	0	0	0	0
1 tsp. olive oil	40	0	0	5	0	0
Total:	1,379	176	77	43	22	2,849
		51%	22%	28%		

DAY 28

Meal/Snack	Calories	Carbs (g)	Protein (g)	Fat (g)	Fiber (g)	Sodium (mg)
BREAKFAST						
2 Turkey Sausage Patties (page 186)	110	0	13	6	0	330
1 whole-grain low-fat waffle	71	14	2	1	1	215
1 Tbsp. maple syrup	52	13	0	0	0	1
1 Tbsp. light whipped butter	35	0	0	3	0	4.5
½ small banana, sliced	46	12	0.5	0	1	5
SNACK						
1 cup strawberries	50	12	1	1	4	2
LUNCH						
1 cup vegetable-beef soup	160	22	8	2	4	900
3 Stoned Wheat Thins crackers	90	15	3	2	2	210
1 cup cucumber sticks	10	2	0	0	0	0
1 Fat-Free Fudgsicle	60	12	2	0	0	40
SNACK						
½ cup mango chunks	54	14	0	0	1	2
DINNER						
1 serving Shrimp Shack Special (page 249)	240	23	25	6	5	660
2 cups salad with butterhead lettuce	20	4	1	0	1	13
½ cup artichoke hearts	38	8	3	0	4	45
1 Tbsp. olive oil and vinegar dressing	120	0	0	14	0	0
1 serving Orange Cheesecake with Glazed Blueberries (page 267)	170	17	12	6	0	230
Total:	**1,326**	**168**	**70.5**	**41**	**23**	**2,657.5**
		51%	21%	28%		

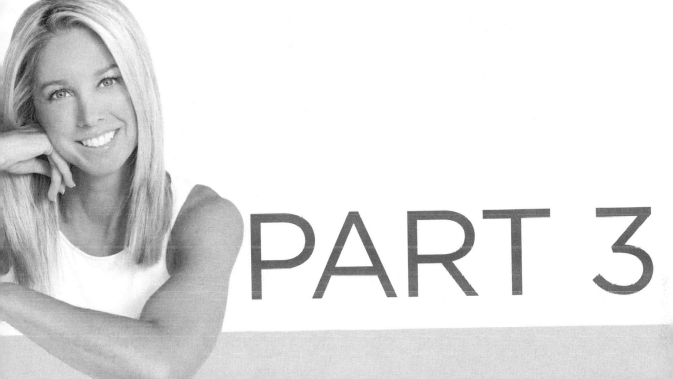

PART 3

The *Eat Carbs,* *Lose Weight* Recipes

9

BREAKFASTS

Get your metabolism humming with these tasty morning dishes

Are you a breakfast eater? If you said yes, then you are already on the road to a more healthful lifestyle and a successful weight loss. In fact, people who avoid breakfast are more likely to be overweight. A wholesome breakfast featuring high-quality carbs balanced with protein and fat ensures that you have the fuel to power on through the morning without succumbing to sugary temptation. Eating the right type of breakfast is the key.

Breakfast is a great time to pack in some fiber. Important for controlling appetite, fiber helps you to feel fuller sooner and keeps you feeling fuller longer. Since you're aiming for 25 to 30 grams a day, get a jump on your total with the first meal of the day.

A great way to go is high-fiber cereal with berries and fat-free milk—a no-brainer. But our recipes will take you beyond the cereal bowl. Soon you'll be enjoying parfaits, smoothies, and savory scrambles.

You'll love our morning favorites—Coffee-Chocolate Waffles, Double-A Applesauce Muffins, Almond Cloud Pancakes with Peaches, all packed with good carbs and fiber. They'll fit into your day as easily as they fit into your diet. Because you are pressed for time, especially in the morning, our recipes are super-easy to prepare. They're family-friendly, too—though we've included several for those occasions when you're eating on your own. Watch for the "Just for You" logo.

DAY 1 BREAKFAST BURRITO

Prep: 8 minutes   Cook: 15 minutes

The red and yellow cherry tomatoes combine with the pale green avocado for a gorgeous salsa. Spiked with lime and cumin, the flavors pop.

CHERRY TOMATO-AVOCADO SALSA

1½	cups quartered firm red and/or yellow cherry tomatoes
½	ripe avocado, finely chopped
1	tablespoon fresh lime juice
¼	teaspoon ground cumin
	Pinch of salt

BURRITOS

4	whole-wheat flour tortillas (7½″ diameter)
½	cup canned fat-free refried beans
4	large eggs
2	tablespoons water
⅛	teaspoon salt
⅛	teaspoon coarsely ground black pepper

To make the salsa: In a small bowl, gently mix together the tomatoes, avocado, lime juice, cumin, and salt. Cover and set aside.

To make the burritos: Warm the tortillas in the microwave or a conventional oven according to the package directions. Cover with foil and keep warm.

Place the beans in a small microwave-safe bowl, cover, and microwave on high power for 45 seconds, or until hot. Keep warm.

In a medium bowl, whisk the eggs, water, salt, and pepper until well blended.

Coat a medium nonstick skillet with cooking spray. Heat over medium heat. Add the eggs and scramble until cooked but still moist.

One at a time, spread each warm tortilla with about 2 tablespoons of the beans and fill with ¼ of the eggs. Top each with about 2 tablespoons salsa, reserving the rest to serve at the table. Roll up the tortillas, folding in the sides. Serve right away, with the remaining salsa.

Makes 4 burritos

Per burrito: 290 calories, 32 g carbohydrates, 13 g protein, 12 g total fat, 210 mg cholesterol, 6 g dietary fiber, 480 mg sodium

COFFEE-CHOCOLATE WAFFLES

Prep: 20 minutes   Cook: 15 minutes

These chocolaty treats pack a healthy wallop of fiber and monounsaturated fats to keep you satisfied for hours.

1½	cups whole-grain pastry flour
½	cup unsweetened cocoa powder
2	teaspoons baking powder
¼	teaspoon baking soda
1	cup 1% milk
½	cup packed light brown sugar
2	teaspoons espresso powder
3	tablespoons light olive oil
3	large egg whites
⅛	teaspoon salt
2	tablespoons mini chocolate chips (optional)
	Maple syrup

In a large bowl, whisk together the flour, cocoa powder, baking powder, and baking soda. Make a well in the center of the flour mixture and add the milk, brown sugar, espresso powder, and oil. Whisk the liquid ingredients together until blended. Whisk in the dry ingredients just until combined.

Preheat a waffle iron for 4 minutes, or according to the manufacturer's instructions. (A drop of water should sizzle and bounce when dropped onto the hot grids.)

Meanwhile, beat the egg whites and salt with an electric mixer at high speed just until they form soft peaks. Fold the whites into the chocolate batter in 3 additions, folding in the chocolate chips with the last addition of whites. Fold just until the mixture is combined.

Spray the heated waffle grids with cooking spray right before using. Add enough batter to almost cover the waffle grids (¾ cup) and cook for 3 to 4 minutes. Repeat with the remaining batter. Serve the waffles with maple syrup.

Makes 5 round waffles

Per waffle: 235 calories, 29 g carbohydrates, 10 g protein, 10 g total fat, 0 mg cholesterol, 5 g dietary fiber, 400 mg sodium

Note: To keep the waffles warm, place them in a single layer on a foil-lined baking sheet in a preheated 250°F oven.

DAY 3 FRUITY GINGER SMOOTHIE

Prep: 10 minutes

Start your meal with a fruity kick. Both mangoes and strawberries are low in calories and high in fiber. When choosing ripe mangoes, look for yellow-green or reddish skin that yields to gentle pressure. You can also buy frozen mango chunks.

1½	**cups cubed mango**
2	**cups strawberries**
1	**tablespoon minced candied ginger**
2	**tablespoons honey**
1	**cup soy milk or 1% milk, chilled**
	Pinch of ground allspice
2	**strawberries (optional)**

In a blender, combine the mango, 2 cups strawberries, ginger, honey, soy milk or milk, and allspice. Process until smooth. Pour the mixture into 2 glasses. Garnish with whole strawberries (if using).

Makes 3 cups

Per 1½ cups: 191 calories, 42 g carbohydrates, 4 g protein, 3 g total fat, 20 mg cholesterol, 4 g dietary fiber, 42 mg sodium

Note: For a frozen smoothie, place the fruit on a baking sheet lined with waxed paper and freeze for 2 hours, or until almost firm. Use as directed in the recipe.

SMOKED SALMON SPREAD DAY 7

Prep: 10 minutes   Stand: 30 minutes

This savory breakfast spread is a perfect brunch entrée. Made ahead, it's also a convenient and portable breakfast.

4	ounces reduced-fat cream cheese
2	ounces smoked salmon, coarsely chopped
1	teaspoon fresh lemon juice
1	tablespoon chopped fresh dill
2	tablespoons coarsely chopped green onions
¼	teaspoon freshly ground black pepper
16	slices thin-sliced pumpernickel bread

Place the cream cheese in a food processor and pulse until smooth, about 15 seconds. Add the salmon, lemon juice, dill, green onions, and pepper. Process until all the ingredients are incorporated, about 15 seconds. Place the cream cheese mixture in a small bowl, cover, and chill for at least half an hour for the flavors to develop. The spread can also be made the day before and chilled overnight.

To serve, spread 1 tablespoon salmon mixture on a slice of pumpernickel bread, cut in half, and place on a serving dish. Repeat with the remaining ingredients.

Makes 1 cup spread

Per 2 tablespoons spread and 2 slices pumpernickel: 134 calories, 20 g carbohydrates, 5 g protein, 4 g total fat, 8 mg cholesterol, 3 g dietary fiber, 311 mg sodium

DAY 8 WHOLE-WHEAT FRENCH TOAST
WITH FRESH STRAWBERRIES

Prep: 10 minutes   Cook: 25 minutes

We packed lots of fiber and energy-boosting carbs into this family-friendly breakfast.

3	tablespoons no-sugar strawberry or raspberry spread
2	cups sliced strawberries
1	large egg
1	large egg white
2/3	cup 1% milk
1½	teaspoons vanilla extract
	Pinch of ground nutmeg
2	tablespoons unsalted butter, divided
8	slices thin-sliced whole-wheat bread

Preheat the oven to 200°F. Place a serving platter in the oven to hold the French toast.

Place the spread in a medium bowl and stir until smooth. Stir in the strawberries. Set aside.

In a pie plate or shallow bowl, beat the egg, egg white, milk, vanilla, and nutmeg with a fork until blended.

Melt 1 tablespoon butter in a large nonstick skillet over medium heat.

Dip a bread slice into the egg mixture, letting it soak briefly on both sides. Place the soaked slice in the skillet; add 1 or 2 more soaked slices.

Cook, turning once, until lightly golden, about 3 minutes per side. Place the cooked French toast in the oven to keep warm. Repeat with the remaining bread slices, adding the remaining 1 tablespoon butter as needed.

Serve the French toast hot with the strawberries.

Makes 4 servings

Per serving: 270 calories, 38 g carbohydrates, 11 g protein, 10 g total fat, 70 mg cholesterol, 4 g dietary fiber, 300 mg sodium

WESTERN SCRAMBLE DAY 9

Prep: 15 minutes   Cook: 25 minutes

Red bell peppers are not only pretty and sweet but also very nutritious and a great source of vitamin C. If you like, boil the potatoes for the scramble the night before. To make prep even easier, chop the onions and bell peppers and wrap them separately. You'll be ready to start your breakfast, and your day.

2	small red- or white-skinned potatoes, cut into ½" cubes
1	tablespoon canola oil
1	medium onion, coarsely chopped
1	medium red bell pepper, coarsely chopped
½	medium green bell pepper, coarsely chopped
½	cup extra-lean ham, finely chopped
2	large eggs
4	large egg whites
2	tablespoons low-fat cottage cheese
½	teaspoon coarsely ground black pepper
	Pinch of salt

Put the potatoes in a medium saucepan. Add cold water to barely cover. Bring to a boil over high heat. Reduce the heat to medium, partially cover, and cook until tender, about 7 minutes. Drain.

Heat the oil in a large nonstick skillet over medium-high heat. Add the onion and bell peppers and cook, stirring often, until tender and lightly golden, about 8 minutes. Stir in the ham and potatoes and cook, stirring often, until just starting to brown, 2 minutes.

In a medium bowl, beat the eggs, egg whites, cottage cheese, black pepper, and salt until well blended.

Pour the egg mixture into the skillet. Reduce the heat to medium and cook, turning often with a heatproof spatula, until just set, about 2 minutes.

Makes 4 servings

Per serving: 170 calories, 14 g carbohydrates, 13 g protein, 7 g total fat, 115 mg cholesterol, 2 g dietary fiber, 400 mg sodium

DAY 10 DOUBLE-A APPLESAUCE MUFFINS

Prep: 16 minutes   Cook: 25 minutes

Make a batch of these to freeze for easy breakfasts and snacks. If you don't have currants—tiny, dried, sweet Zante grapes—substitute dark or golden raisins or snipped dried plums (prunes).

1³⁄₄	cups whole-grain pastry flour
2	teaspoons baking powder
¹⁄₂	teaspoon baking soda
1	teaspoon ground cinnamon
¹⁄₈	teaspoon salt
¹⁄₂	cup fat-free plain yogurt
1	large egg
3	tablespoons dark brown sugar
2	tablespoons canola oil
2	medium Golden Delicious apples, grated
³⁄₄	cup unsweetened applesauce
¹⁄₂	cup currants

Preheat the oven to 375°F. Coat 18 muffin cups with cooking spray. (Don't use paper liners.)

In a large bowl, stir together the flour, baking powder, baking soda, cinnamon, and salt.

In a medium bowl, whisk together the yogurt, egg, brown sugar, and oil until smooth. Stir in the apples, applesauce, and currants.

Pour the apple mixture into the dry ingredients and stir until just blended.

Spoon the batter evenly into the prepared cups, filling them nearly to the top. Bake for 20 to 25 minutes, or until springy to the touch and lightly browned. Turn out onto a wire rack to cool.

Makes 18 muffins

Per muffin: 100 calories, 19 g carbohydrates, 2 g protein, 2 g total fat, 10 mg cholesterol, 3 g dietary fiber, 115 mg sodium

FRUITY OATMEAL

Prep: 7 minutes   Cook: 15 minutes

Serve with cold milk and a touch of honey or brown sugar. This can be made ahead of time and refrigerated in individual containers. To serve, cover and warm in the microwave, adding a little more water or milk if the oatmeal seems too thick.

2	cups 1% milk
1	cup water
1½	cups old-fashioned rolled oats
1	medium Golden Delicious apple, diced
1	ripe medium pear, diced

Bring the milk and water to a boil in a large heavy saucepan (nonstick is great) over high heat. Stir in the oats, reduce the heat to medium-low, and simmer for 2 minutes, stirring occasionally, until the oats start to soften.

Stir in the apple and pear, cover, and simmer for 5 to 7 minutes more, until the oats have softened and the fruit is tender.

Makes 4 cups

Per cup: 200 calories, 37 g carbohydrates, 8 g protein, 3.5 g total fat, 5 mg cholesterol, 5 g dietary fiber, 65 mg sodium

DAY 13 BLT SANDWICH

JUST FOR YOU

Prep: 3 minutes   Cook: 6 minutes

Thought BLTs were on the no-no list? No way! Enjoy this hearty, healthy, and portable egg-and-bacon scramble for breakfast or lunch. It will energize your morning.

2	slices turkey bacon, each cut in half
½	cup egg substitute
	Dash of hot-pepper sauce (optional)
1	whole-wheat pita (6″ diameter), halved crosswise
1	tablespoon light mayonnaise
2	leaves lettuce or 4 leaves spinach
2	tomato slices

In a small nonstick skillet, cook the bacon over medium heat until crisp. Remove from the skillet. Cool briefly and crumble or chop coarsely.

In the same skillet, pour the egg substitute, pepper sauce (if desired), and the bacon. Cook over medium-low heat, stirring often, just until eggs are set. Remove from the heat.

Meanwhile, microwave the pita just until hot, 10 to 15 seconds. Spread the mayonnaise inside the pita, then fill it with the lettuce or spinach and tomato slices.

Spoon the egg mixture into the pita and serve.

Makes 1 sandwich

Per sandwich: 366 calories, 48 g carbohydrates, 21 g protein, 13 g total fat, 32 mg cholesterol, 6 g dietary fiber, 965 mg sodium

BREAKFAST PARFAIT

JUST FOR YOU

DAY 14

Prep: 3 minutes

Use your favorite berries to make this parfait. Strawberries, a good source of fiber and vitamins, are almost always available. But in season go wild with raspberries, blueberries, or blackberries. For a special touch and a bit more crunch, toast the almonds.

¼	cup All-Bran cereal
½	cup sliced strawberries, or other fresh berries of your choice
1	container (6 ounces) light vanilla yogurt
2	tablespoons slivered almonds

In a parfait glass or dessert bowl, sprinkle ½ of the cereal. Top with ½ of the berries and ½ of the yogurt. Sprinkle with the remaining cereal. Spoon on the remaining berries and remaining yogurt. Sprinkle the almonds over the top and enjoy.

Makes 1 parfait

Per parfait: 230 calories, 37 g carbohydrates, 10 g protein, 7 g total fat, 4 mg cholesterol, 10 g dietary fiber, 134 mg sodium

DAY 15 ALMOND CLOUD PANCAKES WITH PEACHES

Prep: 4 minutes   Cook: 30 minutes

Ricotta cheese makes these distinctive pancakes light and tender but also offers a nice serving of protein to balance the carbohydrates.

1½	cups frozen sliced loose-pack peaches
4	teaspoons confectioners' sugar, divided
2	large eggs, separated
	Pinch of salt
1	cup part-skim ricotta
1	teaspoon almond extract
½	cup whole-grain pastry flour
1	teaspoon baking powder
⅓	cup fat-free milk

Arrange the peaches in a single layer on a microwave-safe dish. Cover loosely. Microwave on the defrost setting, rotating once, for 2 minutes. Chop coarsely and place in a small bowl. Mix with 1 teaspoon confectioners' sugar.

Beat the egg whites and salt in a small bowl with an electric mixer on medium speed for 1 minute, or until foamy. Increase the speed to high; gradually add 2 teaspoons confectioners' sugar and beat for 1 minute, or until the peaks hold their shape.

In another bowl, beat the egg yolks, ricotta, and almond extract until blended. Stir in the flour and baking powder, then the milk. Fold in the egg whites.

Heat a nonstick griddle or 2 large nonstick skillets over medium-high heat until a drop of water sizzles and bounces when dropped on the surface. Off the heat, spray the pan with cooking spray right before using. Ladle the batter, a scant ¼ cup per pancake, onto the hot surface. Cook for 2 minutes, or until the bottoms are well browned. (These pancakes are delicate, so make sure they are partially cooked before flipping.) With a nonstick spatula, flip the pancakes and reduce the heat. Cook for about 2 minutes, or until the pancakes are cooked through.

Transfer to plates. Place the remaining 1 teaspoon confectioners' sugar in a fine sieve and dust the pancake tops. Spoon the peaches on the side.

Makes 12 pancakes

Per 3 pancakes: 210 calories, 21 g carbohydrates, 13 g protein, 8 g total fat, 125 mg cholesterol, 1 g dietary fiber, 280 mg sodium

CANADIAN BACON AND VEGETABLE HASH

Prep: 10 minutes   Cook: 30 minutes

This unusual and delightful hash combines turnips, potatoes, leeks, and spinach with Canadian bacon for a satisfying and hearty breakfast.

3	turnips
2	red-skinned potatoes
2	teaspoons extra-virgin olive oil
1	small leek, white and light green part, sliced
1½	cups packed baby spinach, shredded
2	Canadian bacon slices, cut into small cubes
¼	teaspoon salt
¼	teaspoon crushed red pepper (optional)

Scrub the turnips and potatoes but do not peel. Place on a microwave-safe dish. Cover loosely and microwave on high power, rotating once, for 5 to 7 minutes, or until the vegetables yield when squeezed (wear an oven mitt). Remove and set aside until cool enough to handle. Peel the turnips. Cut the turnips and potatoes into small cubes.

Heat the oil in a medium nonstick skillet over medium-high heat. Add the leek; toss and cover. Cook, tossing once, for 2 minutes, or until the leek is softened. Add the spinach; toss and cover. Cook for 1 minute, or until the spinach is wilted.

Add the turnips, potatoes, bacon, salt, and red pepper (if using) to the skillet. Toss the mixture and then press down with a spatula. Cover and cook for 2 minutes. Turn the mixture with the spatula and press down. Cover and cook, flipping the mixture and scraping the pan bottom occasionally, for 8 minutes, or until the vegetables are very soft. Reduce the heat if the mixture is browning too quickly.

Makes 4 servings

Per serving: 100 calories, 16 g carbohydrates, 4 g protein, 3 g total fat, 3 mg cholesterol, 3 g dietary fiber, 320 mg sodium

Note: The hash may be covered and refrigerated for up to 3 days. To reheat, place one serving on a microwave-safe plate and cover loosely. Microwave on medium power for 2 minutes.

DAY 20 — FRUIT-SOY SMOOTHIE

JUST FOR YOU

Prep: 5 minutes

Look for strawberries that have been frozen without sugar. When strawberries are ripe and fresh in the market, wash, hull, dry, and freeze them in zip-top bags.

½	cup low-fat plain soy milk, chilled
½	cup fat-free plain yogurt
¼	banana, sliced
½	cup frozen strawberries
1	tablespoon toasted wheat germ

In a blender, combine the soy milk, yogurt, banana, strawberries, and wheat germ. Process until smooth. Pour into a tall glass.

Makes 1 smoothie

Per smoothie: 236 calories, 39 g carbohydrates, 12 g protein, 4 g total fat, 3 mg cholesterol, 5 g dietary fiber, 111 mg sodium

QUICK APPLE-PECAN WAFFLE

JUST FOR YOU

DAY 22

Prep: 2 minutes   Cook: 3 minutes

This super-easy, super-delicious waffle is one of our favorites. Did you know that research has shown that ordinary cinnamon is anything but? It can control blood pressure and blood sugar, so sprinkle away.

1	whole-grain low-fat frozen toaster waffle
¼	cup unsweetened applesauce
⅓	cup light vanilla yogurt
2	tablespoons coarsely chopped pecans
	Pinch of ground cinnamon

Toast the waffle and transfer to a plate. Spread with the applesauce and spoon the yogurt on top.

Sprinkle with the pecans and dust with cinnamon. Eat right away.

Makes 1 waffle

Per waffle: 198 calories, 30 g carbohydrates, 5 g protein, 6 g total fat, 2 mg cholesterol, 3 g dietary fiber, 259 mg sodium

DAY 23 FRENCH TOAST SOUFFLÉ
WITH MAPLE CREAM TOPPING

Prep: 20 minutes   Cook: 20 minutes

Unlike wimpy white bread, stone-ground whole wheat has the body to stand up to a milk and egg bath without disintegrating. So there's no need to remember to dry out the bread beforehand as with regular French toast.

²/₃	cup whole milk
1	large egg, separated
2	teaspoons vanilla extract
1¼	teaspoons ground cinnamon
3	slices stone-ground whole-wheat bread, cut into small cubes
2	large egg whites
	Pinch of salt
3	teaspoons confectioners' sugar, divided
2	tablespoons reduced-fat cream cheese
1	tablespoon whole milk
½	teaspoon maple extract

Preheat the oven to 375°F. Coat a 7" soufflé dish with cooking spray; set aside.

In a large bowl, beat the whole milk, egg yolk, vanilla, and cinnamon with a fork until blended. Add the bread and stir, pressing with the fork. Set aside for about 5 minutes, pressing occasionally, to break up some of the cubes.

In a small bowl, beat the egg whites and salt with an electric mixer on medium speed for 1 minute, or until foamy. Increase the speed to high, gradually adding 2 teaspoons confectioners' sugar. Beat for 1 minute, or until the peaks hold their shape. Fold into the bread mixture. Spoon into the prepared soufflé dish.

Bake for 15 minutes, or until puffed and golden. (The center will still be soft; for a firmer soufflé, bake an additional 2 to 3 minutes.)

Meanwhile, in a small bowl, whisk the cream cheese, milk, maple extract, and the remaining 1 teaspoon confectioners' sugar until smooth. Drizzle the maple cream on each serving.

Makes 4 servings

Per serving: 150 calories, 17 g carbohydrates, 9 g protein, 5 g total fat, 60 mg cholesterol, 1 g dietary fiber, 260 mg sodium

SAUSAGE AND CHEESE SCONES

Prep: 20 minutes   Cook: 30 minutes

So very British, and so very carb-wise. Make these hearty scones ahead of time and freeze them. Reheat frozen scones for a perfect portion-controlled breakfast. Enjoy with a spot of tea! *Note:* Always keep whole-grain flours in the refrigerator or freezer so they remain fresh.

1½	cups whole-grain pastry flour
½	cup unbleached all-purpose flour
2	teaspoons baking powder
¾	teaspoon salt
½	teaspoon baking soda
½	teaspoon dry mustard
½	teaspoon freshly ground black pepper
3	tablespoons cold unsalted butter, cut into bits
4	turkey breakfast sausage links, crumbled and browned
¾	cup shredded reduced-fat sharp Cheddar cheese
¾	cup reduced-fat buttermilk
1	large egg white, lightly beaten with 1 teaspoon water

Preheat the oven to 400°F. Coat a baking sheet with cooking spray.

In a medium bowl, whisk together the pastry flour, all-purpose flour, baking powder, salt, baking soda, mustard, and pepper. Add the butter and blend with a pastry cutter or 2 knives until the dough is crumbly. Add the sausage and cheese; toss to combine. Add the buttermilk and stir until the dough comes together.

Turn out the dough onto a lightly floured surface. Gently knead for about 30 seconds. Pat the dough into a circle, approximately 8" across and 1" thick.

Transfer the dough to the prepared baking sheet and brush with the egg white mixture. Cut into 10 equal wedges. Pull the wedges apart to separate slightly. Bake for 25 to 30 minutes, or until the scones are lightly browned. Cool slightly and serve.

Makes 10 scones

Per scone: 156 calories, 16 g carbohydrates, 7 g protein, 7 g total fat, 22 mg cholesterol, 2 g dietary fiber, 388 mg sodium

DAY 28 TURKEY SAUSAGE PATTIES

Prep: 12 minutes   Cook: 8 minutes

Preparing these tasty sausage patties is so easy you may want to double the recipe and freeze the extras in a zip-top bag. With these on hand, you'll never miss higher-fat pork sausage.

1	large egg yolk
1	teaspoon extra-virgin olive oil
1	teaspoon rubbed sage
1/2	teaspoon ground paprika
1/2	teaspoon salt
1/4	teaspoon freshly ground black pepper
8	ounces ground turkey breast

In a mixing bowl, combine the egg yolk, oil, sage, paprika, salt, and pepper with a fork. Crumble the turkey into the bowl. With a fork or clean hands, combine thoroughly. Shape into 8 patties; place the patties in a single layer on a work surface. Coat both sides lightly with cooking spray.

Heat a large nonstick skillet over medium-high heat. Place the patties in the skillet. Cook for 3 minutes, or until browned. Flip and cook for about 4 minutes, or until cooked through. (Check by cutting a patty in half.) Reduce the heat if the patties are browning too quickly.

Makes 8 patties

Per 2 patties: 110 calories, 0 g carbohydrates, 13 g protein, 6 g total fat, 90 mg cholesterol, 0 g dietary fiber, 330 mg sodium

Note: The patties may be cooled, packed in a resealable plastic freezer bag, and frozen for up to 6 weeks. To reheat, thaw overnight in the refrigerator and then microwave, loosely covered, on medium power for 1 minute.

10

LUNCHES

These quick, satisfying lunches give you the energy to zip through your afternoon

You'll love these lunches! Imagine being able to have a tuna melt; a veggie burger with cheese; a bowl of zesty, fresh gazpacho with croutons; or a sloppy Joe (with bun!) on a diet. They're all here, a diverse collection of flavors and textures, from hearty, filling soups to crisp, refreshing salads to super-satisfying sandwiches.

For days when you're really pressed, we offer easy suggestions in the menu plan for sandwiches or meals that can be purchased at the deli, from a salad bar, or in the cafeteria. And since lunch is often a solo affair, we have a collection of "Just for You" recipes that come together in minutes.

Planning is the key to keep you on your diet. Since most of us work outside the home, it's often easiest to prepare lunch the night before and pack it to go. This works especially well with our soups. To make life even simpler, you can simmer up the Hearty Herbed Chicken Soup or the Southwestern Corn and Sweet Potato Soup on a weekend. Freeze them in meal-size portions and then tote just what you need.

With these recipes, you won't have to give up the foods that you love to get the perfect balance of energy-packed, high-quality carbs, lean proteins, and healthy fats to keep you stepping pretty until dinner.

DAY 1 COUNTRY GARDEN GAZPACHO
WITH GARLIC CROUTONS

Prep: 15 minutes   Chill: 2 hours   Cook: 8 minutes

Choose the ripest tomatoes for the most luscious gazpacho. The whole-wheat croutons round out the carb portion of this make-ahead lunch, plus they add a delicious, satisfying crunch.

2	large garlic cloves
3	large ripe tomatoes, peeled and cut into chunks
1	medium cucumber, peeled and cut into chunks
½	large red bell pepper, cut into chunks
½	cup chopped sweet white or red onion
1	cup tomato juice
1	tablespoon fresh lemon juice
¼	teaspoon salt
⅛	teaspoon ground red pepper
1	tablespoon extra-virgin olive oil
2	slices whole-wheat bread, cut into ½" cubes

With the food processor running, drop 1 garlic clove through the feed tube and process until finely chopped.

In batches, add the tomatoes, cucumber, bell pepper, and onion; process until pureed. Pour into a large bowl.

Stir in the tomato juice, lemon juice, salt, and red pepper. Cover and refrigerate about 2 hours, until well chilled.

Meanwhile, smash the remaining garlic clove with the flat side of a chef's knife or a meat mallet. Place the garlic and oil in a medium nonstick skillet over medium-low heat. Cook, turning and pressing down on the garlic, until golden, about 4 minutes. Discard the garlic.

Add the bread cubes to the garlic oil and cook, stirring, until browned and crisp, 2 to 3 minutes. Transfer the croutons to a bowl and let cool.

To serve, stir the soup and ladle it into bowls. Top each serving with some of the croutons.

Makes 5 cups

Per 1¼ cups: 130 calories, 21 g carbohydrates, 4 g protein, 4.5 g total fat, 0 mg cholesterol, 4 g dietary fiber, 450 mg sodium

Note: If you want to boost the soup's crunch factor, add ½ cup finely chopped red bell pepper and ½ cup finely chopped cucumber to the finished soup as a garnish.

HUMMUS WITH ROASTED RED PEPPERS   DAY 1

Prep: 20 minutes   Chill: 4 hours   Cook: 20 minutes

Chickpeas are the main attraction in this Middle Eastern spread. Just ½ cup of this tasty snack delivers 6 grams of fiber, so you'll stay hunger free for hours. Serve the hummus with assorted vegetable sticks for dipping or use as a spread for wraps or sandwiches.

2	medium red bell peppers
4	large garlic cloves, unpeeled
1	can (15½ ounces) chickpeas, rinsed and drained
2	tablespoons tahini
2	tablespoons fresh lemon juice
1	tablespoon mild pepper sauce
¼	cup chopped fresh cilantro

Preheat the broiler. Place the peppers on a foil-lined baking sheet. Wrap the garlic in foil and place on the sheet. Broil the peppers 6" from the heat for 15 to 20 minutes, turning until charred on all sides. Broil the garlic for 15 minutes. Transfer the peppers to a paper bag, close, and let stand for 10 minutes.

Set the garlic aside until cool enough to handle, then peel the cloves and finely chop in a food processor. When the peppers are cool enough to handle, peel, core, and seed the peppers. (You should have 1 cup of roasted peppers.) Add the peppers, chickpeas, tahini, lemon juice, and pepper sauce to the food processor and blend until smooth. Add the cilantro and process just until combined. For best flavor, cover and refrigerate for at least 4 hours or up to 3 days.

Makes 2 cups

Per ½ cup: 174 calories, 27 g carbohydrates, 7 g protein, 5 g total fat, 0 mg cholesterol, 6 g dietary fiber, 260 mg sodium

DAY 2 GREEK-STYLE VEGETABLE SALAD

Prep: 20 minutes   Stand: 15 minutes

With a nod to the heart-healthy cuisine enjoyed by our Mediterranean friends, this robust salad is loaded with monounsaturated fats and fiber to suppress those urges to overeat.

2½	tablespoons extra-virgin olive oil
1	tablespoon fresh lemon juice
1	tablespoon red wine vinegar
½	teaspoon dried oregano
½	teaspoon salt
½	teaspoon freshly ground black pepper
2	large ripe tomatoes, cut into chunks
1	can (15½ ounces) chickpeas, rinsed and drained
2	cups chopped hothouse cucumbers
½	cup thinly sliced red onion
½	cup coarsely chopped fresh flat-leaf parsley
10	kalamata olives, pitted and sliced
4	cups torn mixed dark-hued greens, such as escarole and romaine lettuce, or all romaine
4	ounces feta cheese, finely chopped

In a large salad bowl, use a fork to mix the oil, lemon juice, vinegar, oregano, salt, and pepper.

Add the tomatoes, chickpeas, cucumbers, onion, parsley, and olives. Toss to mix well. If you have time, let marinate for 15 minutes.

Add the greens and feta and toss again.

Makes 4 servings

Per serving: 338 calories, 34 g carbohydrates, 12 g protein, 18 g total fat, 25 mg cholesterol, 8 g dietary fiber, 1,040 mg sodium

TURKEY-VEGGIE PITA

JUST FOR YOU

Prep: 7 minutes

These days, the deli counter is filled with different flavors and styles of roast turkey breast. Choose your favorite but be sure to remove any skin before preparing the sandwich. Smoked turkey would be tasty as well.

1	oat-bran pita (6″ diameter), halved crosswise
3	ounces sliced roast turkey breast, skin removed
½	cup shredded green leaf lettuce
¼	avocado, cut into chunks
2	teaspoons grainy Dijon mustard
1	teaspoon vinaigrette salad dressing

Fill the pita halves with the turkey, lettuce, and avocado.

In a cup, mix the mustard and dressing and drizzle over the sandwich halves.

Makes 1 serving

Per serving: 391 calories, 42 g carbohydrates, 33 g protein, 17 g total fat, 71 mg cholesterol, 7 g dietary fiber, 461 mg sodium

DAY 5 SMOKED TURKEY, ARUGULA, AND CRANBERRY WRAP

Prep: 25 minutes   Cook: 12 minutes

Turkey doesn't contain much saturated fat or many calories, yet it is incredibly satisfying. This wrap can be prepared the night before (pack the arugula separately) and wrapped to take for the next day's lunch.

1	tablespoon extra-virgin olive oil
2	onions, thinly sliced
1	jalapeño chile pepper, seeded and finely chopped (wear plastic gloves when handling)
¼	teaspoon chili powder
¼	teaspoon dried oregano
1	pound deli-sliced smoked turkey breast
4	spinach-flavored tortillas (8″ diameter)
½	cup prepared cranberry sauce
1	cup loosely packed arugula leaves

Heat a medium nonstick skillet over medium heat and add the oil. Add the onions, jalapeño, chili powder, and oregano. Cook, stirring occasionally, for 10 to 12 minutes, or until the onions are golden and tender. Remove from the heat and cool for 10 minutes.

Place ¼ of the turkey down the center of each tortilla. Top with 2 tablespoons cranberry sauce, 2 tablespoons onions, and ¼ cup arugula. With the filling facing you horizontally, fold up the bottom of the tortilla over the filling. Fold in the 2 sides and then roll the bottom over the filling to form a package.

Makes 4 wraps

Per wrap: 331 calories, 39 g carbohydrates, 26 g protein, 9 g total fat, 45 mg cholesterol, 4 g dietary fiber, 1,120 mg sodium

SLIM SLOPPY JOES

Prep: 5 minutes   Cook: 25 minutes

The kids will enjoy this classic unadorned, but adults may want to spice it up by topping their sandwiches with chopped sweet onion, pickle slices, or pickled banana peppers. Serve the Sloppy Joe mixture on whole-wheat burger buns (toasted, if desired) and use ½ cup of the beef per serving. This makes enough for two meals, so you could freeze the remainder for later.

12	ounces lean ground beef round or sirloin
1	teaspoon canola oil
1	large green bell pepper, chopped
2	cans (8 ounces each) tomato sauce
⅔	cup frozen corn kernels
2	tablespoons ketchup
1	tablespoon cider vinegar
1	teaspoon sugar
¼	teaspoon freshly ground black pepper

Coat a large nonstick skillet with cooking spray and heat over medium-high heat. Crumble in the beef and cook, stirring often, until it loses its pink color, about 5 minutes. Drain the beef in a colander and wipe out the skillet.

In the same skillet, heat the oil over medium heat. Add the bell pepper and cook, stirring often, until tender, about 3 minutes. Return the beef to the skillet and stir in the tomato sauce, corn, ketchup, vinegar, sugar, and black pepper. Bring just to a boil. Reduce the heat and simmer until lightly thickened, about 10 minutes.

Makes 4 cups

Per ½ cup: 150 calories, 21 g carbohydrates, 12 g protein, 3.5 g total fat, 25 mg cholesterol, 3 g dietary fiber, 470 mg sodium

DAY 7 HEARTY HERBED CHICKEN SOUP

Prep: 20 minutes   Cook: 45 minutes

Chicken is an excellent way to keep your diet steady and predictable. The veggies in this soup add good-for-you carbs to keep your energy level high.

4	skinless, bone-in chicken breast halves, well trimmed (about 2 pounds)
2	large garlic cloves, minced
1	tablespoon chopped fresh thyme
¼	teaspoon freshly ground black pepper
½	teaspoon salt, divided
5	cups chicken broth
1	cup water
3	medium carrots, cut into 1" pieces
2	medium white turnips, peeled and cut into wedges
3	celery stalks with leaves, cut into 1" pieces
2	medium onions, cut into wedges
½	cup chopped fresh flat-leaf parsley

With kitchen shears, cut the chicken breasts in half crosswise.

In a cup, mix the garlic, thyme, pepper, and ¼ teaspoon salt. Rub the mixture all over the chicken and place the chicken in a Dutch oven.

Add the broth, water, carrots, turnips, celery, onions, and the remaining ¼ teaspoon salt. Cover and bring to a boil over high heat. Reduce the heat to low and simmer for about 45 minutes, or until the vegetables are tender and the chicken is no longer pink. Remove the chicken from the soup; cut into bite-size pieces, removing the bones. Return the meat to the pot.

Stir in the parsley and ladle into deep soup bowls.

Makes 12 cups

Per 2 cups: 323 calories, 21 g carbohydrates, 48 g protein, 5 g total fat, 105 mg cholesterol, 5 g dietary fiber, 1,490 mg sodium

AVOCADO QUESADILLA

Prep: 15 minutes   Cook: 10 minutes

Did you know that avocados are really a fruit and a good source of fiber? The most flavorful avocados are the pebbly, dark-skinned Haas variety. They are grown in Mexico and California.

1	ripe avocado, pitted, peeled, and finely chopped
1	medium tomato, chopped
1/4	cup chopped green onions
1	tablespoon chopped fresh cilantro
1	teaspoon finely chopped jalapeño chile pepper (wear plastic gloves when handling)
1/2	teaspoon salt
1	cup shredded reduced-fat Monterey Jack cheese
4	reduced-fat whole-wheat tortillas (8" diameter)

In a small bowl, mix the avocado, tomato, green onions, cilantro, jalapeño, and salt.

Fill 1 tortilla at a time. Sprinkle 1/4 cup of the cheese over half of each tortilla; top with 1/2 cup of the avocado mixture. Fold the tortillas over to form half circles.

Heat a nonstick griddle or 2 large nonstick skillets over medium-high heat until a drop of water sizzles and bounces when dropped on the surface. Off the heat, spray the surface with cooking spray right before using.

Place the tortillas in the pans and press down slightly. Cook for 2 minutes; carefully flip with a nonstick spatula. Continue cooking for 2 minutes. To serve, cut each tortilla in half.

Makes 4 quesadillas

Per quesadilla: 270 calories, 29 g carbohydrates, 12 g protein, 13 g total fat, 15 mg cholesterol, 5 g dietary fiber, 783 mg sodium

DAY 10 SHRIMP AND AVOCADOS WITH CHILES AND LIME

Prep: 25 minutes   Stand: 15 minutes   Cook: 4 minutes

Shrimp are a great low-fat, protein-rich delicacy with a touch of omega-3 fatty acids. Mix them up with the monounsaturated fats found in avocados and olive oil for a power lunch.

1	pound medium shrimp, thawed if frozen, peeled and deveined
½	teaspoon grated lime peel
3	tablespoons fresh lime juice, divided
1	teaspoon ground cumin, divided
½	teaspoon salt, divided
¼	teaspoon freshly ground black pepper
⅛	teaspoon ground red pepper
1	pound ripe tomatoes, cut into ½" chunks
½	cup coarsely chopped sweet white onion
¼	cup + 2 tablespoons coarsely chopped fresh cilantro
2	tablespoons chopped pimiento-stuffed green olives
1–2	tablespoons finely chopped fresh jalapeño chile pepper, with the seeds (wear plastic gloves when handling)
2	tablespoons extra-virgin olive oil
1	ripe avocado, pitted, peeled, and cut into chunks
4	cups mixed greens

Place the shrimp in a medium bowl and add the lime peel, 1 tablespoon lime juice, ½ teaspoon ground cumin, ¼ teaspoon salt, black pepper, and red pepper. Mix well, cover, and set aside while preparing the salad.

In another medium bowl, combine the tomatoes, onion, ¼ cup cilantro, olives, jalapeño, oil, and the remaining 2 tablespoons lime juice, ½ teaspoon cumin, and ¼ teaspoon salt. Mix well. Let stand for 10 to 15 minutes to blend the flavors. Add the avocado and mix gently.

Place the greens in a large shallow bowl and mound the avocado mixture in the center.

Spray a medium nonstick skillet with cooking spray. Warm over medium-high heat. Add the shrimp and cook, turning often, for about 4 minutes, or until just opaque in the thickest part.

Add the shrimp and any pan juices to the salad and sprinkle with the remaining 2 tablespoons cilantro. Serve immediately.

Makes 4 servings

Per serving: 296 calories, 15 g carbohydrates, 27 g protein, 16 g total fat, 170 mg cholesterol, 7 g dietary fiber, 570 mg sodium

PEPPERONI PITA PIZZA DAY 11

Prep: 8 minutes   Cook: 10 minutes

Turkey pepperoni and a whole-wheat pita add flavor to this fun lunch choice.

2	whole-wheat pitas (6" diameter)
1	cup pizza sauce
1	cup shredded part-skim mozzarella cheese
2	ounces sliced turkey pepperoni (about 32 slices)
¼	cup chopped roasted red peppers
4	teaspoons grated Parmesan cheese
1	teaspoon extra-virgin olive oil

Preheat the oven to 400°F. Split the pitas in half to form circles.

Place the pita halves on 2 baking sheets. Spread ¼ cup pizza sauce on each pita half to within ½" of the edge. Sprinkle each half with ¼ cup mozzarella. Arrange pepperoni slices on top of the cheese. Sprinkle each pizza with 1 tablespoon peppers and top with 1 teaspoon Parmesan. Drizzle the oil over the pizzas.

Bake for 10 minutes, or until the cheese is melted. Remove to serving plates and cut into quarters.

Makes 4 pizzas

Per pizza: 241 calories, 27 g carbohydrates, 13 g protein, 9 g total fat, 16 mg cholesterol, 1 g dietary fiber, 701 mg sodium

DAY 13   TORTILLA CRISPS WITH MASHED BEANS AND AVOCADO

Prep: 15 minutes   Cook: 9 minutes

Nothing beats beans for a fiber fix. Make 'em zesty in this flavorful lunch treat. The refried beans and avocado (which is rich in heart-healthy fats) will fill you up and keep your cravings at bay.

4	corn tortillas (6″ diameter)
1	plum tomato, seeded and chopped
½	ripe medium avocado, chopped
2	tablespoons finely chopped red onion
1	tablespoon chopped fresh cilantro
1	teaspoon fresh lime juice
¼	teaspoon salt
½	teaspoon canola oil
1	cup fat-free refried beans
1	teaspoon chili powder
½	teaspoon ground cumin
1	cup shredded romaine lettuce
½	cup shredded reduced-fat Monterey Jack cheese

Preheat the oven to 400°F.

Place the tortillas on a baking sheet and spray lightly with cooking spray. Bake the tortillas for 7 to 8 minutes, turning once, until crisp. Remove from the oven and transfer to 4 serving plates.

Meanwhile, in a medium bowl, combine the tomato, avocado, onion, cilantro, lime juice, and salt.

Heat the oil in a medium nonstick skillet over medium heat. Add the refried beans, chili powder, and cumin and cook, stirring, for 2 to 3 minutes, or until hot.

Spread ¼ cup of the bean mixture over each tortilla. Top each with ¼ cup of the lettuce, ¼ cup of the tomato mixture, and 2 tablespoons cheese.

Makes 4 tostadas

Per tostada: 247 calories, 34 g carbohydrates, 12 g protein, 7 g total fat, 10 mg cholesterol, 9 g dietary fiber, 790 mg sodium

CHUTNEY CHICKEN WRAP

Prep: 10 minutes   Chill: 20 minutes

Chutney is the secret ingredient that pumps up the flavor of these wraps. Brown-baggers can make these the night before, then keep them well-chilled for a satisfying lunch.

2	tablespoons chutney
¼	cup low-fat mayonnaise
4	low-fat tortillas (8″ diameter)
4	large red lettuce leaves
2	cups shredded cooked chicken breast or 8 ounces sliced smoked turkey breast (from the deli)
1	cup finely shredded carrots

Mix the chutney and mayonnaise in a small bowl. If you have time, cover and refrigerate for 20 minutes for the flavors to develop.

Spread a scant 1½ tablespoons of the chutney mixture on each tortilla. Top each with a lettuce leaf, ½ cup chicken or 2 ounces turkey, and ¼ cup carrots. Roll the wraps tightly and cut in half diagonally.

Makes 4 wraps

Per wrap: 269 calories, 30 g carbohydrates, 23 g protein, 6 g total fat, 53 mg cholesterol, 2 g dietary fiber, 471 mg sodium

DAY 16 BAKED POTATO AND BROCCOLI

JUST FOR YOU

Prep: 10 minutes   Cook: 6 minutes

The next time you're baking potatoes, bake an extra to make this filling lunch dish. Then just reheat the potato in the microwave oven and fill as directed. Or you could micro-bake the potato instead. Scrub and poke it in several places with a fork. Microwave on high power for 5 to 7 minutes, until it feels soft when gently squeezed. The potato needs to stand for a minute or two before filling; use that time to micro-cook the broccoli.

1	medium (5- to 6-ounce) russet baking potato, baked or microwaved
¼	cup salsa
¼	cup shredded low-fat Cheddar cheese
2	tablespoons light sour cream
	Ground black pepper, to taste
½	cup grated carrots
1	cup steamed small broccoli florets

Reheat the potato, if necessary, in the microwave. Cut a long slit in the top of the potato and press the ends in toward the center. With a fork, mash the potato pulp slightly. Add the salsa, cheese, sour cream, and pepper to taste, and mash to mix. Mix in the carrots.

Spoon the broccoli into the potato and serve.

Makes 1 serving

Per serving: 229 calories, 33 g carbohydrates, 21 g protein, 6 g total fat, 16 mg cholesterol, 10 g dietary fiber, 504 mg sodium

MEDITERRANEAN TUNA SALAD

Prep: 20 minutes

For a portable lunch, pack this in a plastic container along with a lemon wedge to squeeze over the salad. The chickpeas and veggies add top-quality carbs to keep you going throughout the day.

2	cans (6 ounces each) water-packed tuna, drained
1	can (15½ ounces) chickpeas, rinsed and drained
1	large red bell pepper, coarsely chopped
1	jar (4 ounces) marinated artichoke hearts, rinsed, drained, and coarsely chopped
⅓	cup coarsely chopped sweet red onion
10–12	kalamata olives, pitted and coarsely chopped
3	tablespoons fresh lemon juice
2	tablespoons extra-virgin olive oil
1	large garlic clove, crushed through a press

Place the tuna in a medium bowl and flake with a fork. Add the chickpeas, bell pepper, artichoke hearts, onion, and olives. Toss to mix well. Add the lemon juice, oil, and garlic and toss until well blended.

Makes 6 cups

Per 1½ cups: 330 calories, 26 g carbohydrates, 26 g protein, 14 g total fat, 35 mg cholesterol, 5 g dietary fiber, 790 mg sodium

DAY 18 TUNA MELT

JUST FOR YOU

Prep: 5 minutes   Cook: 3 minutes

With a few healthful adjustments, the lunch-counter-favorite tuna melt now fits easily into your diet plan. The smart carbs and fiber come from the whole-wheat English muffin. You'll never miss all the fat in the original.

½	cup drained and flaked water-packed tuna
1	tablespoon light mayonnaise
	Ground black pepper to taste
	Fresh lemon juice, to taste
1	whole-wheat English muffin, split and toasted
2	slices (¾ ounce each) low-fat American cheese
2	tomato slices
2	sweet white onion slices (optional)

Preheat the broiler or toaster oven.

In a small bowl, mix the tuna, mayonnaise, pepper, and lemon juice to taste. Spread evenly on the toasted muffin halves.

Place the muffin halves on a small baking sheet and top each half with one slice of cheese, tomato, and onion, if using. Broil 4" to 5" from the heat source for 1 to 3 minutes, until the cheese melts. Serve hot.

Makes 1 melt

Per melt: 401 calories, 31 g carbohydrates, 42 g protein, 11 g total fat, 38 mg cholesterol, 5 g dietary fiber, 1,351 mg sodium

BACON AND CLAM CHOWDER   DAY 19

Prep: 30 minutes   Cook: 1 hour

The omega-3 fatty acids in shellfish have a number of benefits, not the least of which may be a reduced risk of depression. If feeling blue triggers your appetite, try a bowl of this colorful soup!

4	teaspoons extra-virgin olive oil
1	large onion, chopped
2	celery stalks, coarsely chopped
2	large red or yellow bell peppers, coarsely chopped
½	teaspoon freshly ground black pepper
3	ounces Canadian bacon, finely chopped
3	garlic cloves, minced
4	teaspoons chopped fresh thyme
3	cups chicken broth
12	ounces new potatoes, cut into ½" chunks
1	can (14½ ounces) diced tomatoes, drained
½	cup dry white wine (optional)
1½	cups water
12	littleneck clams, well scrubbed

Heat the oil in a Dutch oven over medium heat. Add the onion, celery, bell peppers, and black pepper. Stir well, cover, and cook, stirring occasionally, for 12 to 14 minutes, or until the vegetables are tender.

Stir in the Canadian bacon, garlic, and thyme; increase the heat to medium-high and cook and stir for 5 minutes, or until all the juices have evaporated.

Add the broth and potatoes; cover and bring to a boil. Reduce the heat to medium-low and simmer, covered, for 10 minutes, or until the potatoes are tender. Stir in the tomatoes and wine (if using), cover, and simmer for 5 minutes more. Remove from the heat.

Bring the water to a boil in a medium skillet over high heat. Add the clams; reduce the heat to medium, cover, and cook, stirring often, for 8 to 10 minutes, or until the clams open.

With tongs, transfer the clams to a bowl, discarding those that don't open. Line a fine-mesh strainer with damp paper towels. Pour the clam broth through the strainer into a glass measure, leaving any sand behind. Add the broth to the soup. Reheat if necessary.

Remove the clams from their shells and chop coarsely. Add the clams to the soup; reheat briefly, and ladle into bowls.

Makes 6 first-course servings

Per serving: 169 calories, 20 g carbohydrates, 14 g protein, 5 g fat, 25 mg cholesterol, 4 g dietary fiber, 770 mg sodium

DAY 20 SOUTHWESTERN CORN AND SWEET POTATO SOUP

Prep: 20 minutes   Cook: 35 minutes

Interestingly, sweet potatoes are not botanically related to the potato. They are actually members of the morning glory family. With a respectable amount of protein and high levels of fiber and complex carbohydrates, they will keep your appetite in check.

1	tablespoon extra-virgin olive oil
1	large onion, coarsely chopped
1	medium red bell pepper, coarsely chopped
2	celery stalks, finely chopped
1/4	teaspoon salt
1/4	teaspoon freshly ground black pepper
1 1/2	teaspoons ground cumin
1/4	teaspoon dried oregano
1	large sweet potato, peeled and cut into 1/2" chunks
1	package (10 ounces) frozen corn
4	cups chicken broth
1/2	cup medium-hot salsa, plus extra for serving
1/2	ripe avocado, finely chopped
1/2	cup coarsely chopped fresh cilantro (optional)

Warm the oil in a Dutch oven over medium-low heat. Add the onion, bell pepper, celery, salt, and black pepper. Cover and cook, stirring often, for about 10 minutes, or until tender. Stir in the cumin and oregano.

Add the sweet potato, corn, and broth. Cover, increase the heat to medium-high, and bring to a boil. Reduce the heat to medium, cover, and simmer for 12 minutes, or until the sweet potato is tender. Stir in the salsa and simmer, uncovered, for 5 minutes more.

Ladle into bowls and top each with some of the avocado, cilantro (if using), and extra salsa, if you wish.

Makes 8 first-course servings

Per serving: 161 calories, 30 g carbohydrates, 4 g protein, 5 g total fat, 0 mg cholesterol, 5 g dietary fiber, 680 mg sodium

ROASTED VEGGIE SANDWICH   DAY 21

Prep: 20 minutes   Cook: 15 minutes

This recipe is loaded with fiber and monounsaturated fats. A colorful assortment of vegetables with a splash of olive oil will rein in your appetite far into the day.

¼	cup light mayonnaise
2	tablespoons chopped fresh basil
1	tablespoon jarred roasted garlic, chopped
2	teaspoons fresh lemon juice
1	medium red onion, cut into 4 slices
1	large red bell pepper, cut into 8 slices
1	large zucchini, cut on an angle into 8 slices
2	teaspoons extra-virgin olive oil
¼	teaspoon salt
¼	teaspoon freshly ground black pepper
8	slices whole-wheat sourdough bread
¾	cup prepared hummus
1	medium tomato, cut into 8 slices

In a small bowl, combine the mayonnaise, basil, garlic, and lemon juice. Set aside.

Coat a grill rack with cooking spray. Preheat the grill. Brush the slices of onion, bell pepper, and zucchini with the oil. Sprinkle with salt and black pepper.

Place the onion and pepper slices on the rack and grill, turning once, for 10 to 12 minutes, or until the vegetables are well marked and tender. Place the zucchini slices on the rack and grill, turning once, for 6 to 8 minutes, or until marked and tender.

Spread 4 slices of the bread with the hummus and place on a cutting board. Top each with an onion slice separated into rings, 2 bell pepper slices, 2 zucchini slices, and 2 tomato slices. Spread the remaining bread slices with the mayonnaise mixture and place on top of the tomatoes. Cut each sandwich in half to serve.

Makes 4 sandwiches

Per sandwich: 310 calories, 45 g carbohydrates, 11 g protein, 12 g total fat, 5 mg cholesterol, 9 g dietary fiber, 680 mg sodium

Note: The vegetables for this sandwich can be grilled the day before and stored, well wrapped, in the refrigerator until ready to use.

DAY 22   CARROT AND PEA SALAD

Prep: 8 minutes   Cook: 10 minutes

This salad is best served freshly made—otherwise the pear may discolor. To make the salad ahead, prepare it without the pear; gently toss in the pear just prior to serving. To save prep time, buy the carrots already julienned.

	Pinch of salt
2	**cups frozen peas**
1½	**cups julienned carrots**
⅓	**cup reduced-fat sour cream**
¼	**cup thinly sliced green onions**
1	**teaspoon cider vinegar**
¼	**teaspoon dried dillweed**
⅛	**teaspoon coarsely ground black pepper**
1	**ripe medium pear, coarsely chopped**
2	**tablespoons golden raisins**

Bring ½" water to a boil in a medium saucepan. Add the salt and the peas and carrots. Cook, stirring often, for 2 to 3 minutes, or until the peas are heated and the carrots tender. Drain and rinse briefly under cold running water. Drain again.

In a salad bowl, mix the sour cream, green onions, vinegar, dillweed, pepper, and ¼ teaspoon salt. Add the pear, raisins, and the peas and carrots. Stir to mix well.

Makes 4 cups

Per cup: 150 calories, 27 g carbohydrates, 5 g protein, 3 g total fat, 10 mg cholesterol, 6 g dietary fiber, 125 mg sodium

ROMAINE SALAD WITH PITA CRISPS AND SESAME

Prep: 20 minutes   Cook: 15 minutes

The diminutive pine nut is a strong ally in the weight-loss battle. These ivory-colored gems contain the monounsaturated fats and the fiber you need to resist a snack attack. Removing the stubborn nuts from the inside of a pinecone is difficult work, which makes them somewhat expensive—but they're worth it.

2	whole-wheat pitas (6″ diameter)
½	teaspoon dried oregano, divided
3	tablespoons pine nuts
2	teaspoons sesame seeds
2	tablespoons extra-virgin olive oil
5	teaspoons fresh lemon juice
1	small garlic clove, crushed through a press
⅛	teaspoon ground paprika
¼	teaspoon salt
6	cups sliced romaine lettuce
1	cup chopped red and green bell peppers
1	cup whole small radishes
1	cup cucumber chunks
½	cup coarsely chopped fresh flat-leaf parsley
3	green onions, whites sliced ½″ thick and greens sliced 1″ thick

Preheat the oven to 425°F.

Split the pitas in half to form circles. Place the rounds rough side up on a baking sheet and sprinkle with ¼ teaspoon oregano. Place the pine nuts and sesame seeds in a small baking pan or ovenproof skillet.

Bake the pitas for 5 minutes, without turning, until crisp and toasted. Bake the pine nuts and sesame seeds for 10 minutes, stirring twice, until browned. Remove from the oven. Leave the pitas on the baking sheet. Tip the nuts and seeds into a bowl. Let both cool.

When the pitas are cooled, break into rough 1″ chunks.

In the bottom of a large salad bowl, use a fork to mix the oil, lemon juice, garlic, paprika, salt, and the remaining ¼ teaspoon oregano. Add the romaine, bell peppers, radishes, cucumber, parsley, and green onions. Toss to mix well. Add the toasted pitas and the pine nuts and sesame seeds; toss again.

Makes 6 first-course servings

Per serving: 154 calories, 18 g carbohydrates, 5 g protein, 8 g total fat, 0 mg cholesterol, 4 g dietary fiber, 220 mg sodium

DAY 26   VEGGIE SOFT TACO

JUST FOR YOU

Prep: 7 minutes

Fast food that you make yourself is so much fresher and tastier. This appetizing taco is packed with fiber and flavor, not laden with fat and sodium. Plus, it provides 4 veggie servings.

½	cup canned pinto beans, drained and rinsed
½	cup shredded green leaf lettuce
½	cup chopped green or red bell pepper
½	cup chopped broccoli
½	small tomato, chopped
2	tablespoons shredded part-skim mozzarella cheese
2	tablespoons salsa
5	pitted ripe olives, chopped
1	corn tortilla (6″ diameter)

In a medium bowl, mix the beans, lettuce, bell pepper, broccoli, tomato, cheese, salsa, and olives.

Warm the tortilla in a microwave oven according to the package directions. Transfer it to a plate and spoon the bean and vegetable mixture onto one half. Fold the other half over and serve.

Makes 1 taco

Per taco: 273 calories, 41 g carbohydrates, 12 g protein, 8 g total fat, 8 mg cholesterol, 11 g dietary fiber, 809 mg sodium

BROCCOLI AND SUN-DRIED TOMATO QUICK BREAD   DAY 27

Prep: 15 minutes   Cook: 55 minutes

Warm from the oven, slices of this savory loaf go well with a mound of creamy cottage cheese. For a weekday breakfast, store individually wrapped slices in the freezer. Pop into the toaster oven until golden and then spread with a bit of fat-free cream cheese.

1	cup water
1	cup finely chopped broccoli florets
½	cup finely chopped onion
1½	cups whole-grain pastry flour
½	cup soy flour
¼	cup walnut pieces, finely ground
1½	teaspoons baking powder
½	teaspoon baking soda
½	teaspoon salt
1	cup reduced-fat buttermilk
2	large eggs, lightly beaten
2	tablespoons extra-virgin olive oil
1	teaspoon hot-pepper sauce
¼	cup dry-packed sun-dried tomatoes, finely chopped
2	teaspoons finely chopped fresh rosemary

Preheat the oven to 350°F. Coat an 8½" × 4½" nonstick loaf pan with cooking spray; set aside.

Bring the water to a boil in a small saucepan. Add the broccoli and onion. Stir. Cover and boil for 1 minute, or until the broccoli is bright green. Drain, then rinse well with cold water; pat dry.

In a large bowl, combine the pastry flour, soy flour, walnuts, baking powder, baking soda, and salt. Make a well in the center. Add the buttermilk, eggs, oil, and pepper sauce. With a fork, quickly incorporate the wet and dry ingredients; some lumps should remain. Fold in the tomatoes, rosemary, and the reserved broccoli mixture. Spoon into the prepared pan.

Bake for about 45 minutes, or until a tester inserted in the center comes out clean.

Allow to sit for 5 minutes before turning out onto a cooling rack. Cool before slicing.

Makes 12 slices

Per slice: 120 calories, 13 g carbohydrates, 5 g protein, 6 g total fat, 35 mg cholesterol, 2 g dietary fiber, 250 mg sodium

11

DINNERS

Delight your belly and your palette with these hearty, savory evening meals

I'd love for you to kick back, wind down, relax, and really savor your dinner. These recipes are time friendly, but they eat slow, inviting contemplation and respite from a busy day. Set the table, light a few candles, cue up some soothing music—and turn off the TV. Take the time to taste your food and to appreciate the close of the day. Whet your appetite with some of these delicious dishes, such as Red Wine and Beef Soup, Teriyaki Salmon with Scallion-Cucumber Relish, and Lime-Grilled Chicken with Cuban Salsa. Your comfort-food favorites are all here, too, from pasta to meatloaf, from mashed sweet potatoes to turkey chili. Recipes so basic, so down to earth that the whole family will dig in, feel satisfied, and get energized. You'll want to take a walk together after dessert (yes, dessert), instead of collapsing in front of the television or slumping over the computer screen.

These dishes will become instant favorites, and your body will love you for them. They feature a variety of lean proteins: chicken, fish, pork, and even beef. You'll get carbs from whole grains, beans, and vegetables, plus good fats from olive and canola oils. Fat is not a bad word; it adds delicious flavor and texture to foods, and it also helps you to absorb certain vitamins. The recipes also provide fiber to get you to your daily goal.

Take some moments to reflect and relish your dinner. Eating is about more than just feeding your body. It's about joy.

BAKED SPINACH-STUFFED POTATOES   DAY 1

Prep: 10 minutes   Cook: 25 minutes

When you're baking potatoes for dinner, pop a few extra into the oven for this nourishing, soothing dish. In a pinch, you can bake the potatoes in the microwave. Choose potatoes that weigh 5 to 6 ounces. Buy the frozen spinach that is already cut and comes in a bag.

2	medium baking potatoes, baked and cooled
½	cup fat-free ricotta cheese
½	cup frozen cut spinach
⅛	teaspoon salt
2	tablespoons grated Parmesan cheese

Preheat the oven or toaster oven to 425°F.

Cut the potatoes in half lengthwise. Scoop the potato pulp into a medium bowl, leaving a ¼"-thick shell. Place the potato shells in a small baking pan.

Using a potato masher, mash the pulp with the ricotta until fairly smooth. Stir in the spinach and salt. Spoon the mixture into the potato shells and sprinkle with the Parmesan.

Bake until heated through and lightly browned, about 20 to 25 minutes. Serve hot.

Makes 4 servings

Per serving: 100 calories, 16 g carbohydrates, 5 g protein, 1 g total fat, 5 mg cholesterol, 1 g dietary fiber, 160 mg sodium

DAY 2 SAUTÉED ZUCCHINI WITH GARLIC AND PARSLEY

Prep: 10 minutes   Cook: 12 minutes

A combination of yellow summer squash and zucchini makes a colorful dish.

1	tablespoon extra-virgin olive oil
3	garlic cloves, cut into thin slivers
1/4	cup chopped fresh flat-leaf parsley
1/4	teaspoon dried thyme
1/4	teaspoon salt
1/8–1/4	teaspoon crushed red-pepper flakes (optional)
4	cups thin half-moon slices zucchini
1	tablespoon water

Heat the oil in a large nonstick skillet over medium heat. Stir in the garlic and cook, stirring often, until fragrant and just starting to color, 2 to 3 minutes.

Quickly stir in the parsley, thyme, salt, and pepper flakes (if using).

Add the zucchini and water and toss to coat with the garlic and parsley mixture. Cook, stirring frequently, until tender, about 7 minutes.

Makes 4 servings

Per serving: 50 calories, 4 g carbohydrates, 1 g protein, 4 g total fat, 0 mg cholesterol, 1 g dietary fiber, 160 mg sodium

BROWN RICE AND TANGY BEANS   DAY 3

Prep: 15 minutes   Cook: 40 minutes

This hearty side dish not only is high in fiber but also has that magical mix of protein and carbohydrates to keep your energy levels stable and your appetite on an even keel for hours.

$\frac{1}{2}$	cup brown basmati rice
1	tablespoon extra-virgin olive oil
2	teaspoons minced garlic
$\frac{1}{2}$	cup chopped onion
1	teaspoon dried oregano
1	teaspoon ground cumin
$\frac{3}{4}$	teaspoon ground coriander
$\frac{1}{2}$	cup chopped green bell pepper
1	large plum tomato, seeded and chopped
1	tablespoon red wine vinegar
1	can ($15\frac{1}{2}$ ounces) black beans, rinsed and drained
$\frac{1}{3}$	cup water
$\frac{1}{4}$	teaspoon salt
$\frac{1}{8}$	teaspoon freshly ground black pepper

In a medium saucepan, cook the rice according to the package directions. Fluff the rice with a fork.

Meanwhile, heat the oil in another medium saucepan over medium heat. Add the garlic, onion, oregano, cumin, and coriander. Cook, stirring occasionally, for 2 minutes, or until the onion begins to soften. Add the bell pepper and cook for 4 minutes more, or until softened. Stir in the tomato and vinegar and cook for 1 minute. Add the beans, water, salt, and black pepper. Simmer, stirring occasionally, for 5 minutes. Serve over the rice.

Makes 4 servings

Per serving: 208 calories, 40 g carbohydrates, 7 g protein, 5 g total fat, 0 mg cholesterol, 8 g dietary fiber, 600 mg sodium

DAY 4 LIME-GRILLED CHICKEN WITH CUBAN SALSA

Prep: 20 minutes   Stand: 15 minutes   Cook: 12 minutes

If you prefer not to grill the chicken, simply broil it indoors. This has a wonderful fresh taste and appeal, and you can make it as tame or as spicy as you wish.

SALSA

1	can (15½ ounces) black beans, rinsed and drained
1	ripe mango, peeled and finely chopped
3	tablespoons chopped red onion
3	tablespoons fresh lime juice
2	tablespoons chopped fresh cilantro
½	jalapeño chile pepper, finely chopped (optional; wear plastic gloves when handling)

CHICKEN

4	boneless, skinless chicken breast halves
2	teaspoons grated lime peel
2	tablespoons fresh lime juice
2	teaspoons canola oil
½	teaspoon salt
¼	teaspoon freshly ground black pepper

To make the salsa: In a medium bowl, stir together the beans, mango, onion, lime juice, cilantro, and jalapeño (if using). Set aside while grilling the chicken.

To make the chicken: Place the chicken in a shallow dish. Add the lime peel, lime juice, oil, salt, and pepper and rub the mixture into the chicken. Cover and let stand for 15 minutes.

Meanwhile, preheat the grill or broiler. If using the broiler, coat a broiler-pan rack with cooking spray.

Place the chicken on the grill rack or broiler pan. Cook 4" from the heat, turning once, until the chicken is no longer pink in the thickest part, 10 to 12 minutes.

Serve the chicken with the salsa. If desired, slice the chicken into strips to serve.

Makes 4 servings

Per serving: 290 calories, 22 g carbohydrates, 37 g protein, 5 g total fat, 80 mg cholesterol, 5 g dietary fiber, 620 mg sodium

ROASTED ASPARAGUS AND MIXED VEGETABLES

Prep: 10 minutes   **Cook: 15 minutes**

Vegetables on a diet don't have to be dry and dull. Here you'll combine intensely flavored roasted asparagus with limas, corn, cherry tomatoes, and fresh oregano for a carb- and fiber-packed side dish you'll love.

1	pound asparagus, trimmed
4	teaspoons extra-virgin olive oil, divided
2	teaspoons minced garlic
1	package (10 ounces) frozen baby lima beans, thawed
1	can (7 ounces) yellow corn kernels, drained
1	teaspoon chopped fresh oregano
1	cup cherry tomatoes, halved
½	teaspoon salt
¼	teaspoon freshly ground black pepper

Preheat the oven to 400°F. Coat a baking sheet with cooking spray.

Toss the asparagus with 1 teaspoon of the oil in a medium bowl and spread in a single layer on the baking sheet. Roast for 8 to 10 minutes, or until tender. Remove from the oven and cool for 5 minutes. Cut the asparagus into 1" lengths and set aside.

Heat the remaining 3 teaspoons oil in a large nonstick skillet over medium-high heat. Add the garlic and cook for 30 seconds. Add the lima beans, corn, and oregano. Cook, stirring occasionally, for 3 to 4 minutes, or until the lima beans are tender and the corn begins to brown slightly. Stir in the tomatoes and cook for 2 to 3 minutes, or until the tomatoes begin to wilt. Add the asparagus, salt, and pepper and cook for 1 to 2 minutes, until hot.

Makes 4 servings

Per serving: 199 calories, 31 g carbohydrates, 9 g protein, 5 g total fat, 0 mg cholesterol, 8 g dietary fiber, 420 mg sodium

DAY 6 CHICKEN-CASHEW TOSS ON GREENS

Prep: 25 minutes   Cook: 20 minutes

The amount of fat in one cashew seems sinful. Fortunately, most of it is the monounsaturated kind, which means these rich nuggets will diminish your cravings. And because this dish is so high in protein, you won't be tempted to overeat.

12	ounces boneless, skinless chicken breast halves, cut into thin crosswise strips
4	tablespoons reduced-sodium soy sauce, divided
¼–½	teaspoon crushed red-pepper flakes
3	tablespoons raw cashews
2	tablespoons olive or canola oil, divided
5	garlic cloves, slivered
1½	tablespoons slivered fresh ginger
1	large red bell pepper, cut into thin strips
2	medium carrots, cut diagonally into thin slices
4	green onions, diagonally sliced
½	cup orange juice
3	cups shredded iceberg lettuce
3	cups baby spinach

In a medium bowl, mix the chicken, 2 tablespoons soy sauce, and pepper flakes to taste; set aside.

Cook the cashews in a small nonstick skillet over medium heat, stirring often, for 3 to 4 minutes, or until lightly toasted. Tip onto a plate and let cool.

Heat 1 tablespoon oil in a large nonstick skillet over medium-high heat. Add the garlic and ginger and stir-fry for 1 to 2 minutes, or until fragrant and lightly golden. Add the chicken and stir-fry for 3 to 4 minutes, or until no longer pink. Transfer to a clean bowl.

Place the remaining 1 tablespoon oil in the same skillet and heat over medium-high heat. Add the bell pepper and carrots and stir-fry for 3 minutes. Add the green onions and stir-fry for about 2 minutes more, or until the vegetables are crisp-tender.

Return the chicken and any juices to the skillet. Add the orange juice and the remaining 2 tablespoons soy sauce. Bring to a boil, stirring. Let boil for 30 seconds; remove from the heat.

Mix the lettuce and spinach on a large deep platter or in a wide shallow bowl. Spoon the chicken mixture on top. Sprinkle with the cashews.

Makes 4 servings

Per serving: 286 calories, 18 g carbohydrates, 24 g protein, 11 g total fat, 50 mg cholesterol, 4 g dietary fiber, 670 mg sodium

MAPLE-MASHED SWEET POTATOES

Prep: 5 minutes   Cook: 15 minutes

Choose medium sweet potatoes with firm, unblemished skins—they'll have the best flavor.

1	**pound sweet potatoes, peeled and cut into 2″ chunks**
2	**medium carrots, thinly sliced**
2	**tablespoons maple syrup**
	Pinch of ground nutmeg
	Freshly ground black pepper

Place the sweet potatoes and carrots in a medium saucepan. Add 1″ water, cover, and bring to a boil over high heat. Reduce the heat to medium and simmer for 9 to 10 minutes, or until the vegetables are very tender.

Drain in a colander and return to the saucepan. Mash until smooth. Stir in the maple syrup and nutmeg and pepper to taste.

Makes 4 servings

Per serving: 130 calories, 31 g carbohydrates, 2 g protein, 0 g total fat, 0 mg cholesterol, 4 g dietary fiber, 50 mg sodium

DAY 8 BUTTERMILK MASHED SPUDS WITH GARLIC AND LEEKS

Prep: 10 minutes　　　　　　　　Cook: 30 minutes

Mashed potatoes have the distinct advantage of being loaded with complex carbohydrates and fiber as well as having a creamy, rich texture that makes them the ultimate comfort food. They have the nutritional staying power you need to feel satisfied long after you've taken your last bite.

1½	pounds baking potatoes, cut into eighths
1	medium leek, white part only, washed and chopped
2	garlic cloves, sliced
½	cup chicken broth
¾	cup reduced-fat buttermilk
2½	tablespoons butter
¾	teaspoon salt
¼	teaspoon freshly ground black pepper

Place the potatoes in a large saucepan with enough water to cover by 3". Bring to a boil over medium-high heat and cook for 17 to 20 minutes, or until tender. Drain and return to the saucepan. Mash until fairly smooth.

Meanwhile, in a medium saucepan, combine the leek, garlic, and broth. Bring to a boil over medium-high heat, reduce the heat to medium, and simmer for 8 to 10 minutes, or until tender. Drain. Stir in the buttermilk, butter, salt, and pepper. Warm gently over medium heat, stirring often, for 2 minutes, or until the butter melts. Add to the potatoes and stir until well combined.

Makes 4 servings

Per serving: 165 calories, 19 g carbohydrates, 7 g protein, 8 g total fat, 20 mg cholesterol, 5 g dietary fiber, 270 mg sodium

SAUTÉED RED PEPPERS
WITH BALSAMIC VINEGAR AND ALMONDS

Prep: 4 minutes   Cook: 14 minutes

The little bit of sugar added to the peppers balances the acidity of the vinegar. These are delicious hot or cold.

2	tablespoons slivered almonds
1	tablespoon extra-virgin olive oil
3	red bell peppers, cut into ¾" strips
1	teaspoon brown sugar
¼	teaspoon salt
	Pinch of freshly ground black pepper
2	tablespoons balsamic vinegar

Cook the almonds in a large nonstick skillet over medium heat, stirring often, until lightly toasted, about 3 minutes. Tip out onto a plate.

Combine the oil and bell peppers in the same skillet. Cook over medium heat, stirring often, until the peppers start to soften, about 4 minutes.

Sprinkle the peppers with the brown sugar, salt, and pepper and toss well. Continue to cook, stirring often, until the peppers are tender and browned in spots, about 4 minutes more.

Add the vinegar and let bubble for about 1 minute, shaking the pan, until reduced to a glaze. Transfer to a serving dish and sprinkle with the almonds.

Makes 4 servings

Per serving: 90 calories, 8 g carbohydrates, 2 g protein, 6 g total fat, 0 mg cholesterol, 2 g dietary fiber, 150 mg sodium

DAY 9 TROPICAL SALAD WITH BABY GREENS

Prep: 20 minutes

Avocados are one of the best sources of monounsaturated fat you can buy. Just half of one of these buttery beauties delivers 9.7 grams! Mixing avocados with the fiber of mangoes and grapefruit gives you a tropical treat that keeps your cravings controlled for hours.

1	tablespoon extra-virgin olive oil
1	tablespoon dry sherry
1½	teaspoons red wine vinegar
¼	teaspoon salt
⅛	teaspoon freshly ground black pepper
1	large pink grapefruit
4	cups mixed baby greens
1	cup sliced ripe avocado
1	cup sliced mango
2	tablespoons chopped red onion

In a salad bowl, combine the oil, sherry, vinegar, salt, and pepper and mix with a fork.

With a serrated knife, peel the grapefruit, cutting off most but not all of the white pith. Working over a bowl, cut out the fruit from in between the membranes. Add 1½ tablespoons of the grapefruit juice to the dressing and mix well.

Add the greens, avocado, mango, onion, and grapefruit sections to the dressing and toss gently to mix. Serve immediately.

Makes 4 first-course servings

Per serving: 129 calories, 12 g carbohydrates, 2 g protein, 9 g total fat, 0 mg cholesterol, 4 g dietary fiber, 220 mg sodium

STEAK AND BELL PEPPER FAJITAS

Prep: 15 minutes   Stand: 4 hours   Cook: 18 minutes

These zesty fajitas prove that eating right means never having to give up your favorite foods. Here's the nutrition bonus in this savory dish: iron from lean beef, nutrients from bell peppers, and smart carbs and fiber from the tortillas. Olé!

1	tablespoon extra-virgin olive oil
4	garlic cloves, minced
1	teaspoon grated lime peel
2	tablespoons fresh lime juice
1	teaspoon ground cumin
1	pound lean round sirloin tip, trimmed of all visible fat
½	teaspoon salt, divided
1	red bell pepper, cut into ¼" strips
1	green bell pepper, cut into ¼" strips
1	onion, cut into ¼" slices
4	whole-wheat tortillas (8" diameter)
½	cup medium-hot salsa
¼	cup fat-free sour cream

In a resealable plastic bag, combine the oil, garlic, lime peel, lime juice, and cumin. Add the sirloin and toss well to coat. Seal the bag and refrigerate for 4 hours or overnight.

Preheat the grill or broiler. Remove the sirloin from the marinade and sprinkle with ¼ teaspoon salt; reserve the marinade. Grill or broil 4" from the heat for 5 to 6 minutes per side, or until a thermometer inserted in the center registers 145°F for medium-rare. Transfer to a cutting board and cover loosely with foil.

Heat a large nonstick skillet over medium-high heat. Add the red bell pepper, green bell pepper, onion, and any marinade left in the bag from the sirloin. Cook, stirring often, for 8 to 9 minutes, or until the vegetables are softened. Add the remaining ¼ teaspoon salt and stir well.

Warm the tortillas according to the package directions. Thinly slice the sirloin across the grain on a slight angle.

To assemble, place the tortillas on individual plates. Top with the sirloin, vegetables, salsa, and sour cream.

Makes 4 servings

Per serving: 308 calories, 32 g carbohydrates, 29 g protein, 9 g total fat, 70 mg cholesterol, 4 g dietary fiber, 700 mg sodium

DAY 10   BAKED CHICKEN THIGHS WITH CHICKPEAS AND TOMATOES

Prep: 15 minutes   Cook: 1 hour 5 minutes

This dish solves two dinnertime dilemmas. It provides a new, family-pleasing way to cook chicken, and it adds 5 grams of fiber to your daily total.

1	can (15½ ounces) chickpeas, rinsed and drained
1	large tomato, finely chopped
1	large onion, coarsely chopped
2	garlic cloves, minced
½	teaspoon dried oregano
½	teaspoon salt
¼	teaspoon freshly ground black pepper
4	bone-in chicken thighs (1¾ pounds), skinned and trimmed of visible fat
1	tablespoon extra-virgin olive oil
¼	teaspoon ground paprika

Preheat the oven to 375°F.

In a 9" × 9" baking dish, combine the chickpeas, tomato, onion, and garlic. In a cup, mix the oregano, salt, and pepper. Sprinkle ½ teaspoon of the herb mixture over the chickpea mixture and stir to mix.

Rub the remaining herb mixture into the chicken. Arrange the chicken on the chickpea mixture and drizzle all with the oil. Sprinkle the chicken with the paprika.

Cover with foil and bake for 45 minutes. Uncover and bake for 15 to 20 minutes more, until the chicken is cooked through. Serve hot or warm.

Makes 4 servings

Per serving: 240 calories, 25 g carbohydrates, 18 g protein, 7 g total fat, 55 mg cholesterol, 5 g dietary fiber, 590 mg sodium

PORK TENDERLOIN AND VEGETABLE STIR-FRY DAY 11

Prep: 10 minutes   Cook: 15 minutes

Packed with good carbs and vitamins, broccoli is the nutritional hero in this appetizing stir-fry. For the freshest broccoli, look for crisp stalks and tightly closed heads. We often only use the florets, but the stalks shouldn't be discarded. Pare off the tough skin with a small knife and slice them thin. Steam or stir-fry the slices in a little olive oil and season with soy sauce or a splash of lemon.

1	pound pork tenderloin, trimmed of all visible fat
2	tablespoons reduced-sodium soy sauce
1	tablespoon dry sherry
1	tablespoon cornstarch
1	tablespoon toasted sesame oil
3	cups broccoli florets
1	medium carrot, sliced on the diagonal
¼	teaspoon crushed red-pepper flakes
1	tablespoon grated fresh ginger
2	garlic cloves, minced
½	cup orange juice
3	tablespoons hoisin sauce

With a sharp knife, cut the pork into 1½" × ¼" strips and place in a bowl. Add the soy sauce, sherry, and cornstarch; toss to combine.

Heat the oil in a large nonstick skillet over medium-high heat. Add the broccoli, carrot, and pepper flakes. Cook, stirring often, for 3 to 4 minutes. Remove to a plate. Add the ginger and garlic to the pan and cook for 1 minute more.

Stir in the pork and cook for 4 minutes, or until the pork is no longer pink. Add the broccoli mixture to the pan and toss for 1 minute. Add the orange juice and hoisin sauce and bring the mixture to a boil. Cook for 1 minute more, stirring to coat, until the mixture thickens slightly.

Makes 4 servings

Per serving: 267 calories, 16 g carbohydrates, 26 g protein, 10 g total fat, 75 mg cholesterol, 3 g dietary fiber, 580 mg sodium

DAY 11 VEGGIE RICE WITH EGG

Prep: 25 minutes Cook: 47 minutes Stand: 15 minutes

Here's a super example of a smart-carb choice. By cooking brown rice instead of white, you get a carb with the bran, germ, and fiber intact—all lacking in white rice. Adding the vegetables and egg makes this a tasty complement to the stir-fried pork.

²/₃	cup brown basmati rice
2	tablespoons toasted sesame oil, divided
1	large egg, lightly beaten
2	teaspoons grated fresh ginger
1	teaspoon minced garlic
2	green onions, cut into ¼" pieces
4	ounces snow peas, trimmed
½	cup frozen peas and carrots, thawed
3	tablespoons reduced-sodium soy sauce

In a medium saucepan, cook the rice according to the package directions. Fluff the rice with a fork, spread it on a baking sheet, and allow to cool completely, about 15 minutes.

Heat 1 tablespoon oil in a large nonstick skillet over medium-high heat. Add the egg and cook, stirring, for about 2 minutes, or until firm. Transfer to a plate and reserve. Heat the remaining 1 tablespoon oil in the skillet and add the ginger, garlic, green onions, and snow peas. Cook, stirring often, for 2 minutes. Add the rice and peas and carrots; cook for 2 to 3 minutes, or until the vegetables are crisp-tender. Add the soy sauce and cook for 3 to 5 minutes more, or until the rice is heated through. Cut the egg into strips or pieces and add to the rice. Serve.

Makes 4 servings

Per serving: 228 calories, 32 g carbohydrates, 6 g protein, 9 g total fat, 45 mg cholesterol, 4 g dietary fiber, 530 mg sodium

SUPER "BOWLFUL" CHILI

Prep: 20 minutes   Cook: 1 hour 10 minutes

There's no need to avoid carbs when they're as nutritious as sweet potatoes and beans—or as yummy. The beans will help to stabilize your appetite, so you'll be satisfied for the evening. The chipotle chile pepper packs heat—if you prefer a milder brew, leave it out.

1	pound ground turkey breast
1	large onion, chopped
2	red or yellow bell peppers, chopped
4	large garlic cloves, minced
3	tablespoons tomato paste
2	tablespoons chili powder
1	tablespoon ground cumin
1	teaspoon dried oregano
1	teaspoon salt
1	large sweet potato, peeled and cut into ½" cubes
1	can (28 ounces) diced tomatoes
1	can (14 ounces) chicken broth
1	chipotle chile pepper in adobo sauce, minced (optional)
2	cans (15 to 16 ounces each) mixed beans for chili, rinsed and drained
1	zucchini, chopped

In a large soup pot or Dutch oven over medium-high heat, cook the turkey, onion, and bell peppers, stirring frequently, for 8 minutes, or until the turkey is cooked through. Add the garlic, tomato paste, chili powder, cumin, oregano, and salt. Cook, stirring constantly, for 1 minute.

Add the sweet potato, tomatoes (with juice), broth, and chipotle chile (if using). Bring to a boil. Reduce the heat to low, cover, and simmer, stirring occasionally, for 30 minutes.

Stir in the beans and zucchini. Return to a simmer. Cover and simmer, stirring occasionally, for 30 minutes more, or until the flavors are well blended and the vegetables are tender.

Makes 8 servings

Per serving: 227 calories, 29 g carbohydrates, 17 g protein, 5 g total fat, 45 mg cholesterol, 10 g dietary fiber, 680 mg sodium

DAY 13 CHICKEN TENDERS AND BROCCOLI STIR-FRY

Prep: 20 minutes   Cook: 10 minutes

Broccoli is a star member of the cruciferous family. It has a respectable amount of fiber, along with a myriad of other nutrients that earn it top honors among food researchers.

1	large bunch broccoli
½	cup orange juice
2	tablespoons reduced-sodium soy sauce
2	teaspoons cornstarch
2	tablespoons orange marmalade
1	tablespoon canola oil
1	pound chicken tenders, trimmed and cut into 1" pieces
3	green onions, sliced
3	large garlic cloves, minced
1	tablespoon finely chopped fresh ginger
	Pinch of crushed red-pepper flakes
⅓	cup chicken broth
1	red bell pepper, thinly sliced

Cut the broccoli into small florets. Trim and discard about 2" of the tough broccoli stems. Thinly slice the remaining stems.

In a small bowl, combine the orange juice, soy sauce, cornstarch, and marmalade. Stir until blended. Set aside.

Heat the oil in a wok or large nonstick skillet over high heat. Add the chicken and cook, stirring frequently, for 2 to 3 minutes, or until no longer pink. Add the green onions, garlic, ginger, and pepper flakes and stir to combine. With a slotted spoon, remove the chicken to a plate.

Add the broccoli and broth to the pan and reduce the heat to medium. Cover and cook for 2 minutes. Increase the heat to high and add the bell pepper. Cook, stirring frequently, for 2 minutes, or until the broth evaporates and the vegetables are crisp-tender. Stir the sauce and add to the wok along with the chicken. Cook, stirring constantly, for 1 to 2 minutes, or until the sauce thickens and the chicken is hot and cooked through.

Makes 4 servings

Per serving: 351 calories, 25 g carbohydrates, 30 g protein, 15 g total fat, 75 mg cholesterol, 7 g dietary fiber, 710 mg sodium

SESAME NOODLES WITH SALMON

Prep: 20 minutes   Cook: 15 minutes

All fish contain omega-3 fatty acids, but salmon earns top honors. The deeper the color, the more fatty acids salmon has. Chinook salmon has the most.

5	ounces soba noodles
3	cups small broccoli florets
2	large carrots, cut into thin diagonal slices
2	teaspoons toasted sesame oil
1	cup thinly sliced green onions
1	tablespoon finely chopped fresh ginger
1	tablespoon minced garlic
12	ounces skinned salmon fillet, cut crosswise into slices about 1½" long × ⅓" thick
1	teaspoon grated lemon peel
3	tablespoons creamy peanut butter
2	tablespoons reduced-sodium soy sauce
2	tablespoons fresh lemon juice
1½–2	teaspoons Asian chili-and-garlic sauce
1½	cups julienned hothouse cucumber

Bring a large pot of water to a boil over high heat. Add the noodles and cook, stirring often, for 2 minutes. Add the broccoli and carrots and continue cooking, stirring occasionally, for about 4 more minutes, or until the noodles are tender and the vegetables are crisp-tender. Scoop out and reserve about ½ cup cooking liquid. Drain the noodles and vegetables in a colander.

In a large nonstick skillet, combine the oil, green onions, ginger, and garlic. Cook over medium heat, stirring often, for 3 to 4 minutes, or until the green onions are wilted. Transfer half of the mixture to a large salad bowl, leaving the remaining half in the skillet.

Add the salmon to the skillet and sprinkle with the lemon peel. Cook, stirring gently with a spatula, for 4 to 5 minutes, or until just opaque in the thickest part. Remove from the heat.

(*continued*)

With a whisk, mix the peanut butter, soy sauce, lemon juice, and chili sauce into the green onion mixture in the salad bowl. Gradually whisk in 3 to 4 tablespoons of the pasta cooking liquid until creamy.

Add the noodles and vegetables and the cucumber to the peanut butter mixture and toss to mix well. Add the salmon and any pan juices and toss gently. Serve immediately or refrigerate for 1 to 2 hours, until ready to serve. If the salad is too dry, add a little more pasta cooking liquid.

Makes 4 servings

Per serving: 439 calories, 40 g carbohydrates, 28 g protein, 18 g total fat, 50 mg cholesterol, 6 g dietary fiber, 500 mg sodium

RED WINE AND BEEF SOUP

Prep: 20 minutes   Cook: 25 minutes

To slice top round easily, wrap it in plastic wrap and freeze for about 20 minutes, until it just starts to firm up. With only 25 percent of calories from fat, top round is one of the healthiest cuts of beef.

12	ounces well-trimmed lean boneless beef top round
$\frac{1}{2}$	teaspoon salt, divided
$\frac{1}{2}$	teaspoon coarsely ground black pepper
4	cups fat-free beef broth
$\frac{1}{2}$	cup dry red wine (optional)
$\frac{1}{2}$	cup tomato sauce
$\frac{1}{4}$	teaspoon dried thyme
1	tablespoon extra-virgin olive oil
1	medium sweet white onion, halved and thinly sliced
2	green bell peppers, cut into strips
4	garlic cloves, minced
3	tablespoons water, divided
$1\frac{1}{2}$	cups halved cherry tomatoes

Thinly slice the beef on the diagonal into ¼"-thick slices. Cut large pieces in half. Sprinkle with ¼ teaspoon salt and the black pepper. Set aside.

In a large saucepan, stir together the beef broth, wine (if using), tomato sauce, and thyme. Cover and bring to a boil over high heat. Reduce the heat to low and simmer for 10 minutes to blend the flavors.

Meanwhile, warm the oil in a large nonstick skillet over medium-high heat until hot but not smoking. Add half of the beef slices and cook, turning once, for about 2 minutes, or until browned. Transfer to a clean bowl. Cook the remaining beef and transfer to the bowl.

(continued)

Add the onion, bell peppers, garlic, and the remaining ¼ teaspoon salt to the skillet. Toss to mix well and add 2 tablespoons water. Reduce the heat to medium and cook, stirring often, for about 10 minutes, or until the vegetables are tender. If the pan gets dry, add the remaining 1 tablespoon water. Add the tomatoes and cook, stirring often, for about 5 minutes, or until softened.

Add the beef and any accumulated juices to the broth mixture. Stir in the vegetables. Warm through but don't boil.

Makes 8 to 10 cups

Per 2 cups: 230 calories, 15 g carbohydrates, 26 g protein, 7 g total fat, 50 mg cholesterol, 3 g dietary fiber, 670 mg sodium

TERIYAKI SALMON
WITH SCALLION-CUCUMBER RELISH

Prep: 6 minutes   Cook: 12 minutes

Salmon is such a wonderful source of healthful omega-3 fatty acids and it's so easy to cook that you'll want to enjoy it often.

1¼	pounds skinless salmon fillets, in 4 equal portions
1	cup chopped cucumber, preferably hothouse
¼	cup sliced green onions
¼	cup slivered fresh basil leaves
1	tablespoon rice wine vinegar
	Pinch of salt
2	tablespoons prepared teriyaki glaze

Preheat the oven to 375°F. Coat a shallow nonstick baking pan with cooking spray. Rinse the fillets with cold water and pat dry. Place in the pan. Bake for 8 minutes.

Meanwhile, in a bowl, combine the cucumber, green onions, basil, vinegar, and salt; set aside.

Brush the salmon with the teriyaki glaze. Bake for 3 to 4 minutes, or until the salmon is opaque in the center. Serve with the cucumber mixture on the side.

Makes 4 servings

Per serving: 220 calories, 3 g carbohydrates, 29 g protein, 9 g total fat, 80 mg cholesterol, 0 g dietary fiber, 450 mg sodium

DAY 16 MUSHROOMS STUFFED WITH RICE AND GREENS

Prep: 20 minutes   Cook: 35 minutes   Stand: 10 minutes

Although nearly half the calories of hummus come from fat, virtually none of it is saturated. Add olive oil and walnuts and you have a delectable dose of monounsaturated fats to keep you hunger free for hours. Try to use mushrooms that are about 4½" to 5" in diameter.

1	cup brown rice
2	teaspoons extra-virgin olive oil
1	small onion, chopped
4	cups sliced escarole or Swiss chard
2	large garlic cloves, minced
½	cup jarred roasted red peppers, rinsed and chopped
4	large portobello mushrooms, stems discarded
½	cup prepared hummus, preferably basil-flavored
3	plum tomatoes, sliced
¼	cup walnuts, chopped
¼	cup grated Parmesan cheese

Cook the rice according to the package directions.

Preheat the oven to 400°F.

Heat the oil in a medium skillet over medium-low heat. Add the onion and cook, stirring occasionally, for 5 minutes, or until softened. Add the escarole or Swiss chard and garlic. Cook, stirring occasionally, for 5 minutes, or until wilted. Remove from the heat and stir in the rice and peppers.

Place the mushrooms, gill side up, on a rimmed baking sheet. Spread with the hummus and spoon on the rice mixture, spreading it to the edges. Arrange the tomato slices on top and sprinkle with the walnuts and Parmesan. Bake for 25 to 30 minutes, or until the mushrooms are tender. Let stand for 10 minutes before serving.

Makes 4 servings

Per serving: 260 calories, 30 g carbohydrates, 10 g protein, 12 g total fat, 5 mg cholesterol, 7 g dietary fiber, 250 mg sodium

Note: To prevent the mushrooms from becoming waterlogged, remove any sand or dirt with a brush and wipe with damp paper towels instead of rinsing with water.

SAUTÉED GREEN BEANS
WITH CHERRY TOMATOES AND ONION

Prep: 10 minutes   Cook: 19 minutes

Here's a delicious way to prepare an ordinary vegetable. Frozen beans will work, in a pinch. Prettiest is a combo of green and wax beans, along with two different colors of cherry tomatoes.

12	ounces green beans, trimmed and halved
2	teaspoons extra-virgin olive oil
2	cups thinly sliced sweet white onion
2	cups halved cherry tomatoes
¼	teaspoon salt
	Pinch of freshly ground black pepper
1	tablespoon snipped fresh dill

Bring ½" water to a boil in a large deep skillet over high heat. Add the beans and cook, stirring often, for 6 to 8 minutes, or until tender. Drain the beans. Dry the skillet.

In the same skillet, heat the oil over medium heat. Stir in the onion and cook, stirring often, for about 4 minutes, or until tender and lightly browned. Stir in the tomatoes and sprinkle with the salt and pepper. Cook, stirring often, for 2 to 3 minutes, or until the tomatoes begin to collapse and give up their juices.

Add the beans and stir to mix with the tomatoes and onion. Heat through. Stir in the dill and serve hot or at room temperature.

Makes 4 servings

Per serving: 90 calories, 16 g carbohydrates, 3 g protein, 2.5 g total fat, 0 mg cholesterol, 4 g dietary fiber, 160 mg sodium

DAY 18 BROILED BEEF SLICES WITH BANGKOK SALAD

Prep: 20 minutes   Cook: 15 minutes   Stand: 10 minutes

Did you know that beef can be just as low in saturated fat and as good for you as chicken? If you choose cuts that have the word *loin* or *round* in the name, you have a satisfying meal that is just as healthy as chicken.

12	ounces lean boneless beef top round steak, trimmed of all visible fat
1/2	teaspoon crushed red-pepper flakes, divided
1/8	teaspoon salt
3	tablespoons fresh lime juice
2	tablespoons fish sauce
2	tablespoons olive or canola oil
1	tablespoon sugar
1	garlic clove, crushed through a press
6	cups shredded red and green leaf lettuce, romaine, or mixed greens
1	cup sliced cucumber
1/2	cup thinly sliced sweet white onion
1/2	cup thinly sliced radishes
1/2	cup coarsely chopped fresh cilantro
1/4	cup coarsely chopped fresh mint

Preheat the broiler. Line a broiler pan with foil and coat the rack with cooking spray. Rub the steak on both sides with ¼ teaspoon pepper flakes and the salt.

Broil the steak 4" to 6" from the heat, turning once, for 12 to 15 minutes, depending on thickness, until a thermometer inserted in the center registers 145°F for medium-rare. Transfer to a plate.

In a large salad bowl, combine the lime juice, fish sauce, oil, sugar, garlic, and the remaining ¼ teaspoon pepper flakes. Mix with a fork. Spoon 1 tablespoon of the dressing over the steak on the plate; let the steak stand for 10 minutes.

Add the greens, cucumber, onion, radishes, cilantro, and mint to the remaining dressing and toss to mix well. Divide among individual plates.

Cut the steak into thin slices on an angle and arrange on top of the salads. Spoon the steak juices over the top.

Makes 4 servings

Per serving: 223 calories, 11 g carbohydrates, 22 g protein, 11 g total fat, 50 mg cholesterol, 3 g dietary fiber, 735 mg sodium

CHILE AND CORN STRATA

Prep: 10 minutes   Cook: 45 minutes

Make this the night before, cover tightly, and refrigerate to bake the next day. Serve with salsa, if you like.

2	slices whole-wheat bread, toasted and cut into ½" cubes
1	cup frozen corn kernels, thawed and drained
1	can (4 ounces) chopped mild green chiles, drained, or 5 tablespoons chopped mild green chiles
2	large eggs
2	large egg whites
1¼	cups 1% milk
½–1	teaspoon green Tabasco
⅛	teaspoon salt
¼	teaspoon freshly ground black pepper
¾	cup shredded light Cheddar or Monterey Jack cheese

Scatter the bread cubes, corn, and chiles in an 8" × 8" glass baking dish.

In a medium bowl, beat the eggs and egg whites. Beat in the milk, Tabasco, salt, and black pepper until well blended. Pour the mixture evenly over the bread. Cover with foil and refrigerate overnight.

The next day, preheat the oven to 325°F. Bake, covered, for 30 minutes. Remove the foil, sprinkle with the cheese, and bake 15 minutes more, or until the strata is puffed and set and the cheese has melted. Transfer to a wire rack and let stand a few minutes before serving.

Makes 4 servings

Per serving: 200 calories, 20 g carbohydrates, 16 g protein, 8 g total fat, 120 mg cholesterol, 2 g dietary fiber, 120 mg sodium

DAY 20 CURRIED CHICKEN WITH ALMONDS AND CURRANTS

Prep: 35 minutes   Cook: 35 minutes

Skinless chicken breasts give us lean protein, almonds add fiber and crunch, and the whole-wheat flour coating the chicken pumps up the carbs while helping it to brown. Tomatoes add lycopene and moisture, and the curry powder makes this mild dish delish.

¼	cup sliced almonds
4	boneless, skinless chicken breast halves
½	teaspoon salt, divided
2	tablespoons whole-grain pastry flour
1	tablespoon extra-virgin olive oil
1	medium onion, chopped
2	bell peppers, coarsely chopped
2	garlic cloves, minced
1	tablespoon curry powder
½	teaspoon dried thyme
1	can (16 ounces) diced tomatoes
¼	cup dry red wine or chicken broth
3	tablespoons dried currants

Cook the almonds in a small nonstick skillet over medium heat, stirring often, for 3 to 4 minutes, or until lightly toasted. Tip onto a plate and let cool.

Cut the chicken breasts in half crosswise. Season with ¼ teaspoon salt. Lightly coat with the flour, patting off the excess.

Heat the oil in a large pot or Dutch oven over medium heat. Add the chicken and cook for 3 minutes on each side, or until lightly browned but not cooked through. Remove the chicken to a plate.

Add the onion and bell peppers to the pot. Cook, stirring frequently, for 5 minutes, or until softened. Stir in the garlic, curry powder, thyme, and the remaining ¼ teaspoon salt. Cook for 1 minute, stirring constantly. Add the tomatoes (with juice) and wine or broth and bring to a boil. Reduce the heat and simmer for 5 minutes. Stir in the currants.

Return the chicken to the pot, pushing it down into the sauce. Bring to a boil. Reduce the heat and partially cover the pot. Cook for 10 to 15 minutes, or until a thermometer inserted in the thickest portion of a breast registers 160°F and the juices run clear. Sprinkle with the almonds.

Makes 4 servings

Per serving: 305 calories, 22 g carbohydrates, 31 g protein, 9 g total fat, 65 mg cholesterol, 6 g dietary fiber, 510 mg sodium

EXOTIC MUSHROOMS WITH MADEIRA

Prep: 15 minutes   Cook: 20 minutes

Mushrooms are a favorite diet staple because they are low in calories, a good source of fiber, and a beautiful complement to any main dish. They are a healthy bonus to any meal.

1	tablespoon extra-virgin olive oil
½	cup chopped onion
10	ounces sliced white mushrooms
8	ounces shiitake mushrooms, stemmed and halved
6	ounces oyster mushrooms, trimmed and halved
1	teaspoon chopped fresh rosemary
1	tablespoon minced garlic
½	teaspoon salt
⅛	teaspoon freshly ground black pepper
¼	cup Madeira wine or beef broth

Heat the oil in a large nonstick skillet over medium-high heat. Add the onion and cook for 1 minute. Add the white mushrooms, shiitake mushrooms, oyster mushrooms, and rosemary, mounding them in the skillet. Cook for 10 to 12 minutes, stirring occasionally, until the mushrooms give off their liquid and begin to brown. Add the garlic, salt, and pepper and cook for 2 to 3 minutes more, or until the garlic begins to brown. Pour in the wine or broth and cook for 1 to 2 minutes, or until the liquid is evaporated.

Makes 4 servings

Per serving: 115 calories, 12 g carbohydrates, 6 g protein, 3 g total fat, 0 mg cholesterol, 3 g dietary fiber, 310 mg sodium

Note: Instead of buying separate types of mushrooms, you can use 4 or 5 packages of mixed wild or domestic mushrooms.

DAY 21 HERB-ROASTED IDAHO POTATO FRIES

Prep: 5 minutes   Cook: 35 minutes

Nothing satisfies like potatoes, especially these crunchy, browned, herb-crusted potato wedges. They're great with ketchup, fat-free sour cream, or all by themselves.

1	pound small baking potatoes
2	teaspoons extra-virgin olive oil
½	teaspoon dried thyme
½	teaspoon dried rosemary
¼	teaspoon salt
⅛	teaspoon freshly ground black pepper

Preheat the oven to 425°F. Coat a heavy baking sheet with cooking spray.

Cut each potato in half crosswise. Place the halves cut side down on the cutting board and cut each into 4 wedges. Place the potatoes in a mound on the prepared baking sheet.

In a cup, mix the oil, thyme, rosemary, salt, and pepper. Pour over the potato wedges and toss to mix well. Spread the potatoes out on the sheet.

Bake, stirring 2 or 3 times, until tender and lightly browned, about 35 minutes. Serve hot.

Makes 4 servings

Per serving: 110 calories, 21 g carbohydrates, 2 g protein, 2.5 g total fat, 0 mg cholesterol, 2 g dietary fiber, 150 mg sodium

BROILED PLUM TOMATOES PARMESAN

Prep: 8 minutes   Cook: 7 minutes

This satisfying dish reminds us of fun Italian dinners and is packed with lycopene, a powerful antioxidant.

6	large plum tomatoes
1/2	teaspoon dried marjoram
1/4	teaspoon salt
	Large pinch of coarsely ground black pepper
2	teaspoons extra-virgin olive oil
2	tablespoons grated Parmesan cheese

Preheat the broiler.

Cut each tomato in half lengthwise and remove the core. Arrange the halves cut side up on a broiler-pan rack. Sprinkle each half with marjoram, salt, and pepper and drizzle with the oil. Sprinkle evenly with the Parmesan.

Broil 5" to 6" from the heat, until the tomatoes are heated through and the topping is lightly browned and glazed, about 7 minutes. Serve hot.

Makes 4 servings

Per serving: 50 calories, 4 g carbohydrates, 2 g protein, 3.5 g total fat, 0 mg cholesterol, 1 g dietary fiber, 190 mg sodium

DAY 22 TURKEY AND SPINACH BAKED PEPPERS

Prep: 30 minutes   Cook: 1 hour 5 minutes

Some researchers believe that chile peppers can actually cause your body to burn calories and increase metabolism. The peppers are a perfect complement to this deliciously robust meal.

1	large red bell pepper, cut in half lengthwise
1	large yellow bell pepper, cut in half lengthwise
4	ounces turkey sausage, casing removed
½	medium onion, chopped
1	garlic clove, minced
3	cups shredded spinach
2	ounces finely chopped green chiles, rinsed and drained
¼	teaspoon ground cumin
⅛	teaspoon salt
½	cup cooked brown rice
1	tomato, chopped, divided
½	cup shredded hot pepper Jack cheese, divided

Preheat the oven to 350°F. Bring a large pot of water to a boil. Add the peppers to the boiling water and cook for 3 minutes. Drain the peppers.

Cook the sausage in a large nonstick skillet over medium heat, stirring frequently to break up the pieces, for 6 minutes, or until no longer pink. Remove with a slotted spoon to a large bowl. Add the onion to the skillet and cook, stirring frequently, for 6 to 8 minutes, or until golden brown. Stir in the garlic and cook for 1 minute. Add the spinach, chiles, cumin, and salt. Cook, stirring occasionally, for about 5 minutes, or until the spinach wilts. Add to the sausage. Stir in the rice, half of the tomato, and ¼ cup of the cheese.

Fill the pepper halves with the rice mixture. Place in a shallow baking dish. Spoon the remaining tomato over the filling. Cover the dish loosely with foil. Bake for 30 minutes. Uncover and sprinkle with the remaining ¼ cup cheese. Bake for 10 minutes more, or until the cheese melts and the filling is hot.

Makes 4 servings

Per serving: 186 calories, 15 g carbohydrates, 11 g protein, 9 g total fat, 60 mg cholesterol, 3 g dietary fiber, 390 mg sodium

SESAME-CRUSTED CATFISH WITH CREAMY SALSA DAY 23

Prep: 10 minutes   Cook: 15 minutes

Tilapia, orange roughy, cod, or any other mild white-fleshed fish also works well in this simple dinner dish.

1¼	pounds catfish fillets, in 4 equal portions
1	large egg white
1	tablespoon water
¼	teaspoon salt
2	tablespoons sesame seeds, toasted
¾	cup medium or hot salsa
¼	cup fat-free plain yogurt
¼	cup fresh cilantro leaves

Preheat the oven to 375°F. Coat a nonstick baking pan with cooking spray. Rinse the fillets with cold water and pat dry. In a wide bowl, beat the egg white, water, and salt with a fork.

One at a time, dip the fillets into the egg white mixture, shaking off the excess. Place on the prepared pan. Sprinkle the tops and sides of the fillets with the sesame seeds. Bake for 15 minutes, or until the fillets are opaque in the center.

Meanwhile, in a bowl, combine the salsa and yogurt. Serve over the fillets and sprinkle with cilantro.

Makes 4 servings

Per serving: 190 calories, 7 g carbohydrates, 27 g protein, 6 g total fat, 85 mg cholesterol, 2 g dietary fiber, 530 mg sodium

Note: To toast sesame seeds, place them in a dry medium skillet over medium-high heat. Cook, stirring, for about 2 minutes, or until the seeds are golden and start to pop. Once cooled, toasted seeds may be stored in the freezer for several months.

DAY 23 CHILI POTATO WEDGES

Prep: 10 minutes   Cook: 37 minutes

These spiced-up potato wedges are oven-baked, so they're crispy but way low in fat. They're high in energy-boosting carbs, packing 5 grams of fiber per serving. What a dish!

4	baking potatoes, cut lengthwise into 12 wedges each
1½	tablespoons extra-virgin olive oil
1	teaspoon chili powder
1	teaspoon ground cumin
1	teaspoon ground paprika
1	teaspoon dried oregano
¼	teaspoon dried thyme
1	teaspoon salt
⅛	teaspoon ground red pepper

Preheat the oven to 450°F. Coat a baking sheet with cooking spray.

In a large bowl, combine the potatoes and oil. Toss well to coat. In a small bowl, combine the chili powder, cumin, paprika, oregano, thyme, salt, and red pepper. Sprinkle the spice mixture over the potatoes, tossing well to coat.

Arrange the potato wedges in a single layer on the baking sheet. Bake for 20 minutes. Turn the potatoes over and bake for 15 to 17 minutes more, until crisp.

Makes 4 servings

Per serving: 109 calories, 12 g carbohydrates, 5 g protein, 5 g total fat, 0 mg cholesterol, 6 g dietary fiber, 610 mg sodium

VEGETABLE FRITTATA

Prep: 10 minutes   Cook: 20 minutes

You can serve this filling and attractive dish right from the pan.

4	teaspoons extra-virgin olive oil
1	medium onion, halved and thinly sliced
1	medium red bell pepper, cut into thin strips, strips cut in half crosswise
1	medium zucchini, cut into thin half-moon slices
1	cup frozen peas
2	large eggs
4	large egg whites
2	tablespoons water
2	tablespoons grated Parmesan cheese, divided
2	tablespoons slivered fresh basil, divided
$\frac{1}{4}$	teaspoon salt
$\frac{1}{8}$	teaspoon freshly ground black pepper

Preheat the oven to 375°F.

Heat the oil in a large ovenproof nonstick skillet over medium-high heat. (If the skillet handle is not ovenproof, wrap it in heavy-duty foil.)

Add the onion and bell pepper and cook, stirring often, until tender and starting to brown, about 4 minutes. Stir in the zucchini and cook, stirring often, until tender, about 4 minutes.

Add the peas and cook, stirring often, for 2 minutes, until heated through.

Meanwhile, in a medium bowl, beat the eggs, egg whites, water, 1 tablespoon Parmesan, 1 tablespoon basil, salt, and black pepper until well blended.

Pour the egg mixture into the skillet and reduce the heat. Cook, tilting the pan and lifting up the edges of the frittata to allow uncooked egg to flow underneath, until the edges are firm but the center is very soft, 2 to 3 minutes. Sprinkle with the remaining 1 tablespoon Parmesan.

Transfer to the oven and bake about 5 minutes, or until set. Sprinkle with the remaining 1 tablespoon basil. Cut into wedges and serve hot or warm.

Makes 4 servings

Per serving: 150 calories, 9 g carbohydrates, 11 g protein, 8 g total fat, 110 mg cholesterol, 2 g dietary fiber, 320 mg sodium

DAY 25   SPAGHETTI WITH VEGGIES AND TOFU

Prep: 20 minutes   Cook: 16 minutes

Tofu is an excellent source of calcium and meatless protein. Timing is important with this dish. So that the work goes smoothly, put the pasta water on to boil before you start prepping the vegetables. Start cooking the pasta before you begin stir-frying the vegetables.

6	ounces whole-wheat spaghetti, broken in half
2	tablespoons canola oil
2	tablespoons chopped fresh ginger
3	large garlic cloves, minced
8	ounces cremini, baby portobello, or white button mushrooms, sliced
1	medium yellow or red bell pepper, cut into thin strips
1	medium zucchini, cut into thin half-moon slices
1/8	teaspoon salt (optional)
1 1/2	cups thin asparagus cut into 1" pieces
1	cup chicken broth or vegetable broth
8	ounces firm tofu, cut into 1/2" cubes
1	cup thinly sliced green onions
3	tablespoons reduced-sodium soy sauce

Bring a large pot of water to a boil. Add the pasta and cook according to the package directions until tender. Drain. Return to the pot and cover to keep warm.

While the pasta is cooking, heat the oil in a large, heavy, deep skillet over medium heat. Add the ginger and garlic and cook, stirring, until fragrant, about 1 minute.

Add the mushrooms, bell pepper, and zucchini; increase the heat to medium-high. Sprinkle with the salt (if using) and cook, tossing often with 2 spoons, until the vegetables are crisp-tender, about 6 minutes.

Add the asparagus and broth; bring to a boil. Cover and simmer until the asparagus is crisp-tender, 3 to 4 minutes. Stir in the tofu, green onions, and soy sauce and remove from the heat.

Add the tofu-vegetable mixture to the pasta and toss gently to mix.

Makes 4 servings

Per serving: 320 calories, 44 g carbohydrates, 16 g protein, 11 g total fat, 0 mg cholesterol, 7 g dietary fiber, 560 mg sodium

BRAISED CHICKEN DRUMSTICKS

Prep: 20 minutes   Cook: 55 minutes

Simmered in a rich bath of broth, wine, and aromatic vegetables, these savory drumsticks are finished with a fresh sprinkle of chopped parsley and lemon peel. Chickpeas and tomatoes add the good-tasting, good-for-you carbs, rounding out the balance.

2	tablespoons extra-virgin olive oil
8	chicken drumsticks (2 pounds), skin removed
1/2	teaspoon salt, divided
1	medium onion, chopped
2	carrots, chopped
2	celery stalks, chopped
4	garlic cloves, minced
1	can (14 1/2 ounces) diced tomatoes with red peppers (see note)
1	can (15 1/2 ounces) chickpeas, rinsed and drained
1	cup chicken broth or vegetable broth
1/2	cup white wine or chicken broth
1	bay leaf
1/4	cup chopped fresh flat-leaf parsley
1	tablespoon grated lemon peel

Heat the oil in a soup pot or Dutch oven over medium-high heat. Sprinkle the chicken with 1/4 teaspoon salt. Add the chicken to the pot and cook, turning occasionally, for 6 to 8 minutes, or until browned. Remove the chicken to a plate.

Reduce the heat to low and add the onion, carrots, celery, and the remaining 1/4 teaspoon salt. Cover and cook for 8 minutes, or until the vegetables soften. Reserve 1 teaspoon of the garlic; stir the remaining garlic into the pot and cook for 1 minute. Add the tomatoes (with juice), chickpeas, broth, wine or broth, and bay leaf. Return the chicken to the pot. Bring to a boil. Reduce the heat, cover, and simmer for 30 to 35 minutes, or until the chicken is very tender. Remove and discard the bay leaf.

In a small bowl, combine the parsley, lemon peel, and the remaining 1 teaspoon garlic. Serve the chicken sprinkled with the parsley mixture.

Makes 8 servings

Per serving: 276 calories, 18 g carbohydrates, 28 g protein, 9 g total fat, 80 mg cholesterol, 4 g dietary fiber, 670 mg sodium

Note: Contadina makes tomatoes with red peppers. You can also use Italian-seasoned diced tomatoes or something similar.

DAY 26 ROMAINE AND APPLE SALAD WITH BLUE CHEESE

Prep: 20 minutes   Cook: 4 minutes

Walnuts contain numerous compounds that may protect you from heart disease and cancer. Their fiber and monounsaturated fats, mixed with the crunch of fiber in romaine, give this salad staying power.

2	tablespoons walnuts
5	teaspoons cider vinegar
1	tablespoon walnut oil
2	teaspoons honey
1	teaspoon extra-virgin olive oil
1¼	teaspoons salt
¼	teaspoon freshly ground black pepper
¼	cup chopped red onion
3	cups torn romaine lettuce
½	cup finely shredded red cabbage
½	cup shredded carrot
1	medium Granny Smith, Gala, or Golden Delicious apple, thinly sliced, slices cut in half
2	tablespoons crumbled Roquefort or blue cheese

Cook the walnuts in a small nonstick skillet over medium heat, stirring often, for 3 to 4 minutes, or until lightly toasted. Tip onto a plate and let cool. Chop coarsely.

In a salad bowl, combine the vinegar, walnut oil, honey, olive oil, salt, and pepper. Mix with a fork and stir in the onion.

Add the romaine, cabbage, carrot, and apple and toss to mix well. Sprinkle with the cheese and walnuts.

Makes 4 servings

Per serving: 127 calories, 13 g carbohydrates, 2 g protein, 8 g total fat, 3 mg cholesterol, 3 g dietary fiber, 802 mg sodium

Note: Walnut oil is very perishable and must be kept in the refrigerator. Let it come to room temperature before using.

TURKEY MEATLOAF

Prep: 6 minutes   Cook: 1 hour 25 minutes

Look for ground turkey breast to make this updated comfort food. Regular ground turkey often contains some skin, making it higher in fat and calories. Remaining turkey sausages can be wrapped and frozen to use another day.

1½	teaspoons extra-virgin olive oil
1	medium onion, finely chopped
½	cup finely chopped red bell pepper
2	slices whole-wheat bread, torn into small pieces
⅓	cup 1% milk
1	large egg
12	ounces ground turkey breast
4	ounces sweet Italian turkey sausage, casing removed
2	teaspoons poultry seasoning
¼	teaspoon salt
¼	teaspoon freshly ground black pepper
3	tablespoons ketchup

Preheat the oven to 350°F. Coat a 9" × 9" glass baking dish with cooking spray.

Heat the oil in a small nonstick skillet over medium heat. Add the onion and bell pepper and cook, stirring often, until tender, about 6 minutes. Remove from the heat.

Meanwhile, put the bread in a large bowl. With a fork, stir in the milk and egg. Let stand for 5 minutes, until softened, then mash the bread with the fork.

Add the ground turkey, sausage, poultry seasoning, salt, black pepper, and the sautéed onion and bell pepper. Mix gently until just blended. (Mixture will be soft.)

Shape into a free-form loaf in the prepared baking pan. Spoon the ketchup on top and spread gently with a knife.

Bake for 60 to 70 minutes, or until a thermometer inserted into the center of the loaf registers 170°F. Cool for a few minutes before slicing.

Makes 4 servings

Per serving: 290 calories, 15 g carbohydrates, 28 g protein, 13 g total fat, 125 mg cholesterol, 2 g dietary fiber, 565 mg sodium

DAY 27 BALSAMIC-GLAZED FALL VEGETABLES

Prep: 15 minutes   Cook: 30 minutes

This attractive trio of vegetables contains a powerful mix of complex carbohydrates and fiber to prevent those blood sugar dips that make cookies seem so irresistible.

4	turnips, peeled and cut into 8 wedges each
2	cups frozen small white onions, thawed
1	cup baby carrots
1¼	cups chicken broth
2	tablespoons balsamic vinegar
2	tablespoons dark brown sugar
4	teaspoons butter
½	teaspoon ground cumin
¼	teaspoon salt
⅛	teaspoon freshly ground black pepper
2	tablespoons chopped fresh flat-leaf parsley

In a large skillet, combine the turnips, onions, carrots, broth, vinegar, brown sugar, butter, cumin, salt, and pepper. Bring to a boil over medium-high heat, reduce the heat to medium, and simmer, stirring occasionally, for 24 to 25 minutes, or until the liquid evaporates. Continue cooking, stirring often, for 4 to 6 minutes more, or until the vegetables are golden and shiny. Remove from the heat and stir in the parsley.

Makes 4 servings

Per serving: 173 calories, 31 g carbohydrates, 4 g protein, 5 g total fat, 10 mg cholesterol, 6 g dietary fiber, 580 mg sodium

SHRIMP SHACK SPECIAL

Prep: 14 minutes   Cook: 5 minutes

This dish is fun for the whole family, and it's easy. Buy the shrimp already peeled and deveined. If it's frozen, thaw it in a bowl of cold water, drain, and pat dry. The slaw is made with prepared cole slaw mix and a can of beans—and it's a red slaw, made spicy with chili powder and hot sauce. If you prefer not to make the sauce, simply use premade cocktail sauce.

SHRIMP

1	pound peeled and deveined medium shrimp, thawed if frozen
2	tablespoons fresh lemon juice
1	teaspoon hot-pepper sauce
1	teaspoon extra-virgin olive oil
1/8	teaspoon salt (optional)

SLAW

2	tablespoons reduced-fat mayonnaise
2	tablespoons reduced-fat sour cream
1	tablespoon cider vinegar
1	teaspoon chili powder
1/4–1/2	teaspoon hot-pepper sauce
1/8	teaspoon salt
3	cups prepared cole slaw mix
1	can (15 ounces) pinto beans, rinsed and drained

SHRIMP SAUCE

1/4	cup ketchup
1–2	tablespoons prepared white horseradish
1	tablespoon fresh lemon juice

To make the shrimp: Coat a rimmed baking sheet with cooking spray. Place the shrimp in a mound on the pan and mix with the lemon juice, pepper sauce, oil, and salt (if using). Spread out on the pan. Let stand for 10 minutes while preparing the slaw and the sauce.

(continued)

Preheat the broiler. Broil the shrimp 3" to 4" from the heat until pink and just opaque in the thickest part, about 5 minutes.

To make the slaw: In a salad bowl, mix together the mayonnaise, sour cream, vinegar, chili powder, pepper sauce, and salt. Add the cole slaw mix and beans and toss to mix well.

To make the sauce: In a small bowl, mix together the ketchup, horseradish, and lemon juice.

Serve the shrimp with the sauce and the slaw.

Makes 4 servings

Per serving: 240 calories, 23 g carbohydrates, 25 g protein, 6 g total fat, 155 mg cholesterol, 5 g dietary fiber, 660 mg sodium

12

SNACKS AND DESSERTS

Follow a balanced diet, and all foods—even chocolate—can help you lose weight

Snacks and desserts are in our meal plan because dieting should not mean deprivation. If it does, you won't stick with it. It's that simple.

Snacks are vital to a healthful, calorie-conscious lifestyle. Eating five times a day, three meals and two snacks, every 4 hours or so, will keep your blood sugar at an even keel and hold your cravings way down. If you plan your snacks (and desserts), and they are based on healthful carbs that satisfy, you can avoid unplanned snack attacks. Forbidding sweet, or any, food is simply not realistic, and it can only strengthen your cravings. Instead of avoiding, indulge wisely.

On this plan, every day you will treat yourself with a small serving of your favorite foods—the stuff you crave the most—chocolate, crispy or chewy cookies, cakes. Throughout the menu, you'll find size-sensible daily indulgences. You might get pudding for a snack, or a fruit crisp or a piece of cake after dinner for dessert. Having your dessert (instead of craving it) puts you in control, not the other way around such as when sweets whisper (or yell) to you from the kitchen, urging you to come on down and party.

Our desserts and snacks are planned into your diet as an integral part of our healthful plan. They incorporate whole grains and sweet fruits, all good carbs that will ease your appetite and satisfy you. So eat up —you'll still lose weight.

DAY 4 PECAN CRISPS

Prep: 20 minutes   Cook: 12 minutes

Pecans contain a good amount of fiber, and most of their fat is monounsaturated. That means these tasty nuts will help control your appetite long after you've eaten the last tasty crumb.

¾	cup whole pecans
1½	cups whole-grain pastry flour
¼	cup cornstarch
¼	teaspoon salt
1¼	cups confectioners' sugar, divided
5	tablespoons butter
2	tablespoons safflower or light olive oil
2	tablespoons reduced-fat sour cream
2	teaspoons vanilla extract

Preheat the oven to 350°F.

Place the pecans on paper towels. Microwave on high power for 1½ to 2 minutes, or until heated and fragrant. Place in a food processor while still warm and process with pulses just until finely chopped. (Some small pieces may remain.) Add the flour, cornstarch, and salt and process with pulses until combined. Scrape out onto a sheet of waxed paper. Do not wipe out the bowl.

Add ¾ cup confectioners' sugar to the food processor. Cut the butter into ½" pieces and scatter over the sugar. Process until the butter is cut into small pieces. Add the oil, sour cream, and vanilla and process for 1 minute, or until creamy. Add the dry ingredients and pulse just until combined, scraping down the side of the processor bowl as needed.

Using a rounded measuring teaspoonful of dough for each cookie, roll ¾" balls and place on a baking sheet 1" apart. Bake for 10 to 12 minutes, or until golden on the bottom. Remove from the pans to a sheet of waxed paper. While the cookies are still warm, spoon the remaining ½ cup confectioners' sugar into a sieve and sprinkle evenly over the tops of the cookies. Let cool and store airtight for up to 1 week or freeze for up to 1 month.

Makes about 36 cookies

Per cookie: 63 calories, 6 g carbohydrates, 1 g protein, 4 g total fat, 5 mg cholesterol, 6 g dietary fiber, 0 mg sodium

PINEAPPLE MEXICALI

Prep: 10 minutes   Stand: 15 minutes   Chill: 30 minutes

Pineapple and strawberries offer a delicious way to indulge your sweet tooth without saturated fat and sugar.

2	cups quartered strawberries
1	tablespoon brown sugar
4	cups fresh pineapple cut into ½" chunks
¼	cup chopped fresh cilantro
¼	teaspoon ground cinnamon
⅛	teaspoon ground cumin
¼	teaspoon freshly ground black pepper

Mix the strawberries and brown sugar in a serving bowl. Let stand for 15 minutes to let the juices flow.

Add the pineapple, cilantro, cinnamon, cumin, and pepper to the strawberries and stir gently to mix. Cover and chill for at least 30 minutes, or until ready to serve.

Makes 6 to 8 servings

Per serving: 74 calories, 19 g carbohydrates, 1 g protein, 0 g total fat, 0 mg cholesterol, 3 g dietary fiber, 2 mg sodium

DAY 12   GLAZED PEAR SNACK CAKE

Prep: 20 minutes   Cook: 40 minutes

Choose fragrant, thin-skinned pears that yield to gentle pressure for this cake.

1¾	cups whole-grain pastry flour
1½	teaspoons baking powder
½	teaspoon baking soda
¾	teaspoon ground nutmeg
⅛	teaspoon ground cloves
¼	teaspoon salt
½	cup sugar
1	large egg
1	large egg white
3	tablespoons canola oil
¾	cup reduced-fat buttermilk or fat-free plain yogurt
1	teaspoon vanilla extract
2	ripe medium pears, peeled and cut into ½" chunks
1	teaspoon apple jelly

Preheat the oven to 350°F. Coat a 9" × 9" baking pan with cooking spray.

In a large bowl, stir together the flour, baking powder, baking soda, nutmeg, cloves, and salt.

In a medium bowl, whisk the sugar, egg, egg white, and oil until smooth. Whisk in the buttermilk or yogurt and the vanilla. Stir in the pears.

Pour the wet ingredients into the dry and stir just until blended. (The batter will be very soft.) Scrape into the prepared pan.

Bake for 35 to 40 minutes, or until the cake is springy to the touch and shrinks from the sides and a toothpick inserted into the center comes out clean. Let cool 30 minutes on a wire rack. Spoon the apple jelly on top and spread it gently with a pastry brush. Cut into squares and serve the cake warm or cool.

Makes 12 servings

Per serving: 140 calories, 24 g carbohydrates, 3 g protein, 4.5 g total fat, 20 mg cholesterol, 2 g dietary fiber, 190 mg sodium

FRUIT KEBABS WITH HONEY-MINT SAUCE   DAY 13

Prep: 10 minutes

Vary the fruit according to taste and the season. You could try chunks of papaya, mango, honeydew melon, or watermelon or thick slices of banana.

KEBABS

3	juice-packed canned pineapple rings (reserve juice)
1	kiwifruit
12	cantaloupe chunks (1½")
8	small strawberries

SAUCE

½	cup fat-free plain yogurt
1	tablespoon honey
1	tablespoon pineapple juice (from pineapple rings)
1½	teaspoons chopped fresh mint leaves
	Pinch of ground cinnamon

To make the skewers: Cut each pineapple ring into 4 pieces. Peel the kiwi, cut into 4 wedges, and halve each wedge crosswise. Thread the fruit onto four 10" to 12" wooden skewers, using 3 cantaloupe chunks, 3 pineapple pieces, 2 kiwi pieces, and 2 whole strawberries per skewer.

To make the sauce: In a small bowl, mix the yogurt, honey, pineapple juice, mint, and cinnamon. Serve as a dipping sauce with the skewers.

Makes 4 servings

Per serving: 100 calories, 23 g carbohydrates, 2 g protein, 0 g total fat, 0 mg cholesterol, 1 g dietary fiber, 30 mg sodium

DAY 14 PEACH MELBA

Prep: 8 minutes   Cook: 30 minutes

A fresh, light, and easy dessert that's also good for you. Each serving contains 2 grams of fiber to add to your daily total.

4	ripe medium peaches
2	teaspoons sugar
1	tablespoon unsalted butter, cut into 8 pieces
4	teaspoons no-sugar raspberry spread
	Mint sprigs (optional)

Preheat the oven to 450°F.

Cut each peach in half and remove the pit. Place the halves cut side up in an 11" × 8" glass baking dish.

Sprinkle each peach half with ¼ teaspoon sugar and dot with a piece of butter. Bake until glazed and very tender, 25 to 30 minutes. Remove from the oven and let cool a few minutes.

To serve, spoon ½ teaspoon of the raspberry spread into each peach half. Place 2 peach halves on each of 4 dessert plates and garnish each with a mint sprig (if using).

Makes 4 servings

Per serving: 90 calories, 16 g carbohydrates, 1 g protein, 3 g total fat, 10 mg cholesterol, 2 g dietary fiber, 0 mg sodium

MIXED-BERRY COBBLER
DAY 17

Prep: 10 minutes   Cook: 30 minutes

Berries topped with a dark brown sugar crumble make a sweet and simply satisfying dessert. You could use all one kind of berry if you prefer. It's especially good with super-healthy blueberries.

2	tablespoons whole-grain pastry flour
1	tablespoon dark brown sugar
1	tablespoon cold unsalted butter
1	package (12 ounces) frozen mixed berries
2	tablespoons granulated sugar
1	tablespoon cornstarch
1	teaspoon fresh lemon juice

Preheat the oven to 375°F. Place six 4-ounce ramekins or custard cups in a baking pan.

Whisk the flour and brown sugar in a small bowl. Cut the butter into small pieces, add to the bowl, and rub with your fingers until crumbly.

In a medium bowl, combine the berries, granulated sugar, cornstarch, and lemon juice. Toss to mix. Spoon ½ cup of the berry mixture into each ramekin. Sprinkle each with ½ tablespoon of the crumble dough.

Bake until the topping is golden and the berries are bubbly, about 30 minutes.

Makes 6 cobblers

Per cobbler: 83 calories, 16 g carbohydrates, 1 g protein, 2 g total fat, 5 mg cholesterol, 3 g dietary fiber, 1 mg sodium

DAY 18 TROPICAL AMBROSIA

Prep: 3 minutes   Chill: 20 minutes

Kiwifruit adds a new touch to this old-fashioned favorite, along with fiber and plenty of vitamins. Choose fruit that feels just soft when gently pressed, and use a vegetable peeler to remove the fuzzy brown skin.

⅓	cup light vanilla or lemon yogurt
2	tablespoons shredded coconut
2	kiwis, peeled and sliced
1	cup fresh pineapple chunks
1	medium banana, sliced
	Mint sprigs (optional)

Mix the yogurt and coconut in a small bowl, cover, and chill for 20 minutes for the flavors to develop.

In a medium bowl, mix the kiwis, pineapple, and banana. Gently stir in the yogurt mixture. Serve garnished with mint sprigs (if using).

Makes 3 cups

Per ¾ cup: 89 calories, 20 g carbohydrates, 2 g protein, 1 g total fat, 0 mg cholesterol, 3 g dietary fiber, 13 mg sodium

SAUTÉED BANANAS WITH SPICED YOGURT TOPPING DAY 19

Prep: 6 minutes   Cook: 9 minutes

This is best made with firm yellow bananas. They should not be green or they won't have full flavor, and they shouldn't be speckled with brown or they'll be too soft. This is our light take on the classic dessert Bananas Foster.

TOPPING

²/₃	cup light vanilla yogurt
	Pinch of ground cinnamon
	Pinch of ground ginger
	Pinch of ground nutmeg

BANANAS

4	small ripe bananas
1	tablespoon unsalted butter
1	tablespoon dark brown sugar
2	tablespoons orange juice

To make the topping: In a small bowl, mix the yogurt, cinnamon, ginger, and nutmeg.

To make the bananas: Peel the bananas and cut them in half crosswise and then lengthwise to make 16 pieces. Cut out any brown spots.

Melt the butter in a large nonstick skillet over medium heat. Add the bananas cut side down and cook without turning for 3 to 4 minutes, or until golden. Turn, sprinkle with the brown sugar, and cook for 1 minute. Drizzle the orange juice into the pan and over the bananas. Cook, shaking the pan to mix the orange juice with the pan drippings, for 1 to 2 minutes more, until the bananas are lightly browned on the underside.

With a spatula, remove the bananas from the pan, placing 4 pieces each on 4 dessert plates. Spoon the pan juices over and top each with some of the spiced yogurt. Serve right away.

Makes 4 servings

Per serving: 120 calories, 24 g carbohydrates, 2 g protein, 3 g total fat, 10 mg cholesterol, 2 g dietary fiber, 15 mg sodium

DAY 22 ORANGE-SCENTED CORNMEAL CAKE
WITH FRESH BERRIES

Prep: 25 minutes   Cook: 25 minutes

Olive oil makes this dessert luxuriously rich and adds a healthy dash of monounsaturated fats. You'll feel full hours after you've laid down your fork. This cake is best served the day it is made.

CAKE

³/₄	cup whole-grain pastry flour
¼	cup cornmeal
1	teaspoon baking powder
¼	teaspoon baking soda
¼	teaspoon salt
⅓	cup + 1 tablespoon sugar, divided
3	tablespoons extra-virgin olive oil
½	cup fat-free plain yogurt
2	large eggs
1	tablespoon grated orange peel
2	tablespoons orange juice
¼	teaspoon ground cinnamon

BERRIES

1	cup blackberries
1	tablespoon sugar
1	tablespoon orange juice
1	cup blueberries
1	cup raspberries

To make the cake: Preheat the oven to 350°F. Coat a 9" springform pan with cooking spray.

In a small bowl, combine the flour, cornmeal, baking powder, baking soda, and salt.

In a large bowl, combine ⅓ cup sugar and the oil. Using an electric mixer on high speed, beat for 2 minutes. Add the yogurt, eggs, orange peel, and orange juice. Beat for 1 minute. Add the dry ingredients and beat until blended. Pour the batter into the prepared pan.

In a small bowl, combine the remaining 1 tablespoon sugar and the cinnamon. Sprinkle over the batter. Bake for 20 to 25 minutes, or until a wooden pick inserted in the center comes out clean. Transfer to a wire rack and let cool.

To make the berries: In a food processor or blender, puree ¾ cup of the blackberries, the sugar, and the orange juice until smooth. Strain the puree through a sieve into a small bowl; discard the seeds. Cut the cake into wedges. Spoon the berry sauce over the wedges and sprinkle with the blueberries, raspberries, and the remaining blackberries.

Makes 8 servings

Per serving: 189 calories, 30 g carbohydrates, 4 g protein, 7 g total fat, 55 mg cholesterol, 3 g dietary fiber, 200 mg sodium

Note: When you use an electric mixer to beat citrus peel into a batter, a lot of the peel can cling to the beaters. So be sure to scrape any peel from the beaters back into the batter.

DAY 23 APPLE CRUMBLE WITH OAT CRUST

Prep: 15 minutes   Cook: 45 minutes

Leaving the skins on the apples provides fiber and vitamins, so this dessert is not only good tasting but also good for you.

½	cup old-fashioned rolled oats
2	tablespoons whole-grain pastry flour
3	tablespoons dark brown sugar, divided
½	teaspoon ground cinnamon
4	teaspoons cold unsalted butter, cut into small pieces
3	medium Golden Delicious apples, cut into thin wedges
2	tablespoons water
1	tablespoon fresh lemon juice

Preheat the oven to 350°F.

In a medium bowl, combine the oats, flour, 2 tablespoons brown sugar, and the cinnamon. Mix with a fork, crumbling the lumps of sugar. Add the butter and work it in with your fingers until the mixture begins to form clumps.

Put the apples in a 9" glass pie plate. Add the water, lemon juice, and the remaining 1 tablespoon brown sugar and toss to mix. Sprinkle the oat mixture evenly over the apples.

Bake until the topping is golden and the apples are tender, about 45 minutes. Serve warm.

Makes 4 servings

Per serving: 170 calories, 32 g carbohydrates, 2 g protein, 4.5 g total fat, 10 mg cholesterol, 3 g dietary fiber, 5 mg sodium

BANANA NUT BREAD

Prep: 13 minutes   Cook: 50 minutes

This tastes best if allowed to stand for a day after baking so the flavor can develop. The mashed bananas need not be totally smooth; a few lumps are fine.

2	cups whole-grain pastry flour
2	teaspoons baking powder
½	teaspoon baking soda
1	teaspoon ground cinnamon
¼	teaspoon salt
½	cup sugar
1	large egg
3	tablespoons canola oil
1	cup mashed overripe bananas (about 2 medium bananas)
½	cup light vanilla yogurt
1	teaspoon vanilla extract

Preheat the oven to 350°F. Line an 8" × 4" loaf pan with foil, letting the ends hang over. Coat the foil with cooking spray.

In a large bowl, combine the flour, baking powder, baking soda, cinnamon, and salt.

In a medium bowl, whisk the sugar, egg, and oil until well blended. Whisk in the bananas, yogurt, and vanilla.

Pour the wet ingredients into the dry and stir just until blended. Scrape into the prepared pan.

Bake for 45 to 50 minutes, or until the loaf has shrunk from the sides of the pan and a wooden pick inserted into the center comes out clean. Transfer to a wire rack and let cool for 30 minutes. Using the foil, lift the cake out of the pan. Carefully peel off the foil and let the cake cool completely on the rack.

Makes 12 slices

Per slice: 140 calories, 25 g carbohydrates, 3 g protein, 4 g total fat, 20 mg cholesterol, 2 g dietary fiber, 190 mg sodium

DAY 24 PEARS BAKED IN RUM CREAM SAUCE

Prep: 14 minutes   Cook: 25 minutes

For variety, replace the pears with ripe summer peaches, autumn baking apples, or late-spring strawberries—they're all wonderful drenched with the rum cream. The baking time will vary depending upon the type of fruit. Pears are very nutritious—each one contains about 25 grams of carbohydrate and 4 grams of fiber.

1	teaspoon cornstarch
	Pinch of salt
3	teaspoons brown sugar, divided
³⁄₄	cup whole milk
1	large egg, lightly beaten
³⁄₄	teaspoon rum extract
2	ripe but firm pears, sliced

Preheat the oven to 425°F. Coat a 7" round baking dish with cooking spray.

In a small saucepan, combine the cornstarch, salt, and 2 teaspoons brown sugar; mix with a whisk. In a measuring cup, combine the milk and egg. Whisking constantly, gradually add the liquid to the dry mixture. Whisk over medium-low heat for about 3 minutes, or until the mixture bubbles and thickens. Remove from the heat. Whisk in the rum extract.

Place the pears in the prepared baking dish and cover with the rum cream. Bake for about 15 minutes, or until the edges bubble. Spoon into dessert dishes. Sprinkle with the remaining 1 teaspoon brown sugar.

Makes 4 servings

Per serving: 110 calories, 19 g carbohydrates, 4 g protein, 3 g total fat, 55 mg cholesterol, 2 g dietary fiber, 75 mg sodium

MEXICALI-SPICED ALMONDS   DAY 25

Prep: 5 minutes   Cook: 8 minutes

Be sure to purchase the slivered almonds that look like tiny sticks for this snack. The thinner sliced almonds would burn before the spice coating was toasted.

¾	teaspoon chili powder
1½	teaspoons sugar
1	egg white
2	tablespoons water
2	bags (2¼ ounces each) slivered almonds (about 1 cup)

Preheat the oven to 350°F. Coat a baking sheet with cooking spray.

In a small bowl, combine the chili powder and sugar. In another bowl, beat the egg white and water with a fork. Add the almonds to the whites; toss to coat. Drain through a colander to remove excess liquid. Scatter the almonds on the baking sheet. Sprinkle with the spice mixture. Toss to coat. Spread out in a single layer.

Bake for 8 minutes. Stir the almonds and spread them out. Bake for about 7 to 8 minutes, stirring occasionally, until the almonds are golden brown. Remove to a cooling rack. Store in a tin in a cool spot for up to 2 weeks.

Makes about 1 cup

Per 2 tablespoons: 110 calories, 4 g carbohydrates, 4 g protein, 9 g total fat, 0 mg cholesterol, 2 g dietary fiber, 10 mg sodium

DAY 26 GINGERED PUMPKIN PUDDING

Prep: 10 minutes   Cook: 35 minutes

Keep some canned pumpkin, a good source of vitamin A, on the shelf year-round for this satisfying treat.

1	cup canned pumpkin
³/₄	cup whole milk
1	large egg, lightly beaten
1	tablespoon light brown sugar
³/₄	teaspoon orange or lemon extract
1	teaspoon grated fresh ginger
¹/₄	teaspoon ground cinnamon
	Pinch of salt
4	teaspoons whipped reduced-fat cream cheese

Preheat the oven to 350°F. Coat four 6-ounce custard cups with cooking spray; set on a sturdy baking sheet.

In a medium bowl, whisk together the pumpkin, milk, egg, brown sugar, extract, ginger, cinnamon, and salt. Pour into the custard cups. Bake for 30 to 35 minutes, or until a knife inserted in the center of a pudding comes out clean.

Serve warm or chilled, topped with a dollop of the cream cheese.

Makes 4 servings

Per serving: 90 calories, 11 g carbohydrates, 4 g protein, 3.5 g total fat, 60 mg cholesterol, 2 g dietary fiber, 200 mg sodium

ORANGE CHEESECAKE WITH GLAZED BLUEBERRIES   DAY 28

Prep: 20 minutes   Cook: 1 hour 10 minutes

If you'd like to feel decadent and virtuous at the same time, savor a slice of this sublime cheesecake.

4	large egg whites
	Pinch of salt
6	tablespoons confectioners' sugar, divided
1¼	cups part-skim ricotta cheese
4	ounces fat-free cream cheese, softened
2	large egg yolks
2	teaspoons orange extract
1	tablespoon cornstarch
1	teaspoon light brown sugar
⅛	teaspoon ground cinnamon
4–5	tablespoons cold water
1	cup frozen loose-pack blueberries, thawed

Preheat the oven to 300°F. Coat an 8" springform pan with cooking spray; place on a baking sheet.

Combine the egg whites and salt in a medium bowl. Beat with an electric mixer on medium speed for 1 minute, or until foamy. Increase the speed to high and gradually add 3 tablespoons confectioners' sugar, beating for 1 minute, or until the peaks hold their shape.

In a large bowl, beat the ricotta and cream cheese until smooth. Add the remaining 3 tablespoons confectioners' sugar, egg yolks, and orange extract. Beat until smooth.

Fold the whites into the cheese mixture. Pour the batter into the prepared pan. Cover loosely with foil. Bake for 1 hour, or until a tester inserted into the center comes out clean. Transfer to a wire rack and remove the foil. Cool to room temperature.

(continued)

In a small saucepan, whisk together the cornstarch, brown sugar, and cinnamon. Whisk in 4 tablespoons water. Add the blueberries and any accumulated juice. Cook, stirring constantly and smashing some of the blueberries with the back of a spoon, over medium heat for 3 to 4 minutes, or until the juices are clear and thickened. Cool to room temperature.

If the blueberry topping is too thick to spread easily, mix in up to 1 tablespoon water. Starting at the center of the cheesecake, spoon and spread the blueberry topping over the cheesecake. Refrigerate for several hours to chill.

Makes 6 servings

Per serving: 170 calories, 17 g carbohydrates, 12 g protein, 6 g total fat, 90 mg cholesterol, 0 g dietary fiber, 230 mg sodium

INDEX

Note: <u>Underscored</u> page references indicate boxed text.

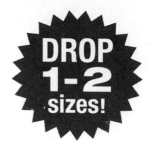
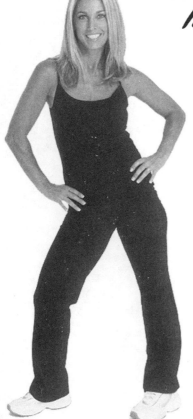
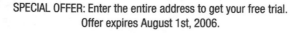